first place
4 health

holiday bible study

light & healthy
holidays

Published by Gospel Light
Ventura, California, U.S.A.
www.gospellight.com
Printed in the U.S.A.

Caution: The information contained in this book is intended to be solely for informational and educational purposes. It is assumed that the First Place 4 Health participant will consult a medical or health professional before beginning this or any other weight-loss or physical fitness program.

Light and healthy holidays six-week holiday devotional.
p. cm.
Includes bibliographical references and index.
ISBN 978-0-8307-4673-6 (trade paper : alk. paper)
1. Holidays—Meditations. 2. Holidays—Prayers and devotions.
3. Holidays—Miscellanea. 4. Health—Religious aspects—Christianity.
I. Gospel Light Publications (Firm)
BV4897.A1L54 2008
242'.2—dc22
2008031530

Rights for publishing this book outside the U.S.A. or in non-English
languages are administered by Gospel Light Worldwide, an international
not-for-profit ministry. For additional information, please visit
www.glww.org, email info@glww.org, or write to Gospel Light Worldwide,
1957 Eastman Avenue, Ventura, CA 93003, U.S.A.

contents

introduction

But seek first his kingdom and his righteousness,
and all these things will be given to you as well.
MATTHEW 6:33

This book is not the typical First Place 4 Health Bible study. Instead, it is a special devotional tool to help you stay on course through the holidays, when many temptations come your way. The Thanksgiving and Christmas holidays can be very busy with many social events, shopping expeditions and church activities that make it difficult to remain faithful to your commitment to living healthy. This book was written to provide order in the hectic holiday season without being a burden on your time. It will give you inspiration for each day and also challenge you to stay on course by daily applying the truths at the core of First Place 4 Health.

One Scripture verse is featured each week, and the daily devotionals use that verse as the reference. The devotionals are holiday-related and give insight and encouragement to maintain balance during the holidays. A prayer and a journaling suggestion follow each reading. A journal page has also been provided for each day to write out your prayers, thoughts and questions.

Holiday Helps and menus for Thanksgiving, Christmas and New Year's Day follow the six weeks of devotional readings. Holiday Helps are valuable tips and suggestions for staying healthy spiritually, mentally, emotionally and physically through the holiday season. Recipes for additional holiday favorites are included with the menus.

Also included at the back of *Light and Healthy Holidays* are weekly prayer partner forms and Live It Trackers. Fill out the weekly prayer partner forms and put them into a basket during your group meeting. After the meeting, you will draw out a prayer partner request form, and this will be your prayer partner for the week. The Live It Tracker is for you to complete at home and turn in to your leader at your weekly meetings.

If you have a plan, you can remain consistent in practicing the spiritual, mental, emotional and physical disciplines you have begun in First Place 4 Health—even through the holidays!

My goals for this holiday season are:

Spiritual: _____

_____

_____

_____

_____

_____

_____

_____

Mental: _____

_____

_____

_____

_____

_____

_____

Emotional: _____

_____

_____

_____

_____

_____

_____

_____

_____

Physical: _____

_____

_____

_____

_____

_____

_____

_____

My strategies for reaching those goals are:

Spiritual: _____

_____

_____

_____

_____

_____

_____

Mental: _____

_____

_____

_____

_____

_____

Emotional: _____

_____

_____

_____

_____

_____

Physical: _____

_____

_____

_____

_____

_____

May the next six weeks take you on a joyful journey toward complete wholeness and health! Here's to the journey!

giving thanks

SCRIPTURE MEMORY VERSE
*Give thanks in all circumstances
for this is God's will for you in Christ Jesus.*
1 THESSALONIANS 5:18

A THANKFUL HEART

Day 1

by Carole Lewis

The Thanksgiving season is a nostalgic time of year for me. My dad went home to be with the Lord just a week before Thanksgiving in 1976. I was 34 years old and had never fixed a holiday meal before, but we had our entire family to our home for Thanksgiving dinner. That became our tradition until just a few years ago when we started going to our daughter Lisa's home for the day.

On Thanksgiving night 2001, our daughter Shari went home to be with the Lord after being struck by a drunk driver while standing behind the family car in the driveway of her in-laws' house, talking to her mother-in-law.

You might wonder how I am able to endure Thanksgiving when sad memories surround the day. Making this verse a part of my life is the reason I can not only endure the day but also enjoy it as well. You see, this verse in 1 Thessalonians tells us to be thankful *in* all circumstances—not *for* all circumstances.

How can I be thankful in the circumstance of never going to my parents' home again for a holiday? Well, our children learned the art of hospitality at an early age. They learned how to set the table and be gracious to those who came to our home for Thanksgiving and Christmas. The lessons they learned all those years ago have helped them as they now carry on our traditions in their own homes. Our daughter Lisa is a great cook like her daddy and is able to make all his Thanksgiving recipes exactly as he did for years. She is so good that she and our daughter-in-law, Lisa, prepare all the meals for our First Place 4 Health Wellness Weeks each year.

How can I be thankful when I think about Thanksgiving without our precious Shari? Well, God has done some great and mighty things for our family in the years since Shari's homegoing. All three of their daughters have grown into lovely young women. Cara, who is 25, graduated from college and married Michael. They now have a baby boy named Luke. Christen is 21 and a student at Texas A & M University. Amanda is 19 and a student at Sam Houston State University. God brought a wonderful Christian woman into their daddy, Jeff's, life a couple of years after Shari died and they were married in September 2007.

Probably the thing I will be most thankful for this Thanksgiving season is that my husband, Johnny, is still here after being diagnosed with stage-4 prostate cancer in 1997. Yes, we battle cancer every day, but our quality of life is good and our God is good. This Thanksgiving will be a wonderful day with the family we love.

Yes, I love this verse so much, I wrote an entire book about it called *A Thankful Heart*!

Dear Lord, thank You for always bringing good from the circumstances of life that have the potential to destroy us. It is only because of Jesus and the Holy Spirit who lives inside us that we are able to walk on water, as Peter did, instead of perishing in the storm (see Matthew 14:22-33).

Journal: Is there something going on in your life right now that you can give thanks *in*, but not *for*? Write about this situation now and know that if you give thanks, God will take you to the other side of the circumstance in power and victory.

CHOOSING THANKFULNESS
by Elizabeth Crews

In 2005, I had the awesome privilege of writing the First Place 4 Health Bible study *Choosing Thankfulness*. The study was intended to be a companion for Carole Lewis's book *A Thankful Heart*, and Carole and I worked on these writings simultaneously. During the writing process, Carole and I talked together via telephone several times a week; however, most of our conversations had nothing to do with what we were writing.

Instead of talking about thankfulness, we often ended up comparing notes on how the enemy was trying to thwart our plans and sabotage our work! It was almost as if Satan were saying, "You two ladies think you can write about being thankful in all circumstances? Well, I've got some special circumstances for you. Let's see if you can practice what you preach." Each week, the enemy's efforts increased. Before long it was almost comical to watch his overkill tactics. But even though Satan was persistent in his efforts, God was faithful to His Word! We were not tempted beyond what we could bear (see 1 Corinthians 10:13), and both of us were convinced that the Lord's hand was on us as we wrote these important words. Praise God that the Spirit in us was stronger than any weaponry the enemy tried to use against us. When complete, both works became a tribute to God's faithfulness and love—a reason for thankfulness no matter what our circumstance.

As part of the research I was doing for *Choosing Thankfulness*, I began to read about the benefits of keeping a thankfulness journal. I was surprised to learn that doing something so simple promised to produce such positive results, and I decided that it was a practice I would begin to incorporate into my own spiritual disciplines. I purchased a composition book and began listing five things I was thankful for each morning and five things I was thankful for each night. At first I was skeptical—and fearful that I would not have enough thanksgiving to write 10 entries each day for the next month. But at the end of the month I was amazed: On many days, I had written down more than 10 things I was thankful for! More than that, I could clearly see God active and working in my life through the simple "Thank You for . . ." sentences I wrote each day.

Three years later, the keeping of a thankfulness journal is an essential part of my daily quiet time with God. And as I have thanked God in all circumstances, I have had more and more reasons to give Him thanks and praise. Each Thanksgiving Day, since I began recording my thankfulness entries on a daily basis, I have taken the time to reread my words. What an awesome God we have! Every day is Thanksgiving Day when we make the decision to keep God first in all things and honor Him by giving Him thanks no matter what our circumstances.

Thank You, Lord, for Your faithfulness and love. No matter what
situation or circumstances I find myself in, I know that You are near.
You hear my prayers and see my distress and come to my rescue.
You are such an awesome God! Today I choose to live a lifestyle
characterized by thankfulness.

Journal: Are you keeping a thankfulness journal? If not, begin the practice today! Write five things in the morning and five in the evening about God's thankfulness and love—and then make a decision to continue the practice of giving thanks in all circumstances until this time next year.

OVERINDULGING IN THANKFULNESS
by Judy Marshall

Before I matured in Christ through First Place 4 Health, I viewed all holidays from the fridge and pantry doors. All my plans revolved around the bountiful spread of the family's favorites on the table—the richest of foods containing thousands of calories with practically no nutritional value. (You know the ones—those we think we cannot possibly live or celebrate without!)

Today, most of those foods are hardly missed at my table, or they have been converted into healthier recipes for family and guests. Through the years with First Place 4 Health, my family has also developed new tastes that have led to new traditional favorites. I find it exciting to shop in the vegetable section and to select from the variety of fresh and colorful fall fruits and vegetables. I scan current magazines and cookbooks to find new and interesting recipes to turn into healthy dishes, and look forward to sharing recipes with other First Place 4 Health members.

When our extended family gets together for Thanksgiving and Christmas, I bring the traditional layered salad, squash casserole and a to-die-for chocolate dessert—all because years ago I volunteered to bring these "legal" dishes so that I wouldn't starve to death while others were overindulging. Today they are requested, expected and gone at the end of the meal!

One of my nieces began the tradition of the Thankful Box, which she and her daughter made together. During our time together, each of us writes on a card what we are thankful for this year. Then after the meal, both past and current cards are displayed on a table for all to read, seeing God's goodness and continued blessings in our extended family over the years. What a treat (right up there with the to-die-for chocolate dessert!). With our focus on God and our responsibility to live balanced and healthy lives even during the holidays, we can see His provision for us and experience the holiday season with a thankful heart. We can always take time to overindulge in thankfulness, which has no calories or added weight—but what blessings it brings!

Lord, may I always be grateful for Your abundance of blessings in my life.
Thank You for the fall bounty of fresh produce and healthy holiday fare.

Journal: Create a "Thankful ABC" entry today. List something you're thankful for that begins with each letter of the alphabet (for example: Almighty God in my life; Beautiful sunset . . .).

GOD IN CONTROL
by Martha Rogers

When I first heard the word "malignant" after a biopsy, I was anything but thankful. First came fear, then anger. I had been doing everything right through First Place 4 Health with my diet and exercise, so why had this disease struck me? After venting my anger toward God, I began to think of everything that might come because of this diagnosis. My mother had just finished her chemotherapy treatments, and I did not want to suffer like she had.

Surgery was scheduled for the following week, and as I prepared, I couldn't stop asking, *Why me?* The answer came back very clearly: "Why *not* you?" Some of the memory verses I had memorized in First Place 4 Health entered my mind and brought great comfort.

However, the morning of my surgery I read through Philippians and Thessalonians for my Bible study lesson, and the topic on giving thanks didn't really interest me. I didn't feel like giving thanks. But then I began to pray, and God showed me that He was still in control. I knew that nothing I could do would change the outcome of what happened in the operating room. At that moment, I gave the cancer completely to Him. What a peace and joy filled my heart! I prayed with thanksgiving that He had shown me the way to peace. I realized I could give thanks to God in any and all circumstances and the result would be His will for my life.

I had such a remarkable recovery! The doctor attributed it to my good health because of First Place 4 Health and my attitude of victory, but I give all the credit to God, who has a purpose for my life and has showed me how to give thanks. And although the cancer returned five years later, I was ready for whatever God planned because I remembered this verse and let it be my testimony again.

It's been well over five years since the second surgery, and I am cancer-free. That is His will and purpose for my life at this time. If the cancer returns, it is part of His will, and I will never cease to praise Him for all He has done for me. I know that no matter what the circumstances or problems in our lives, God already knows them.

Thank You, Father, for all You have done for us. Show us how to fulfill Your will for our lives through whatever may come our way.

Journal: Make a list of the blessings that God has given to you in the past year, and then thank Him for them.

_____

_____

_____

_____

_____

_____

_____

_____

_____

_____

_____

_____

_____

_____

_____

_____

THANKFUL IN HINDSIGHT
by Dee Matthews

Day 5

I was sitting in a Bible study one morning in Rio de Janeiro, listening to the teacher speak about being thankful for everything. I remember thinking that I was not thankful that my son, Robbie, had so many difficult bouts with asthma. He was just three when we moved to Brazil and we made many frightening trips to the hospital, including one when he almost died during the first month we were there.

I remember thinking that there was no way I could be thankful for the way Robbie suffered. I was discouraged that I could not figure out what was causing the sudden attacks and often felt that the school where he attended was feeding him the wrong foods. He was sick almost every weekend.

Looking back on those years, I realize that I had much to be thankful for in the circumstance of Robbie's asthma. While we were still in the hotel prior to Robbie's first hospitalization, someone in the restaurant told me they knew of a pediatrician who had returned to Rio that month. She was an asthma specialist, and she was willing to treat children for any reason. Ultimately, we called her one night when Robbie was ill. She came to the hotel, checked him over, picked him up and drove him to the hospital in her car. She gave him excellent care and became a wonderful friend, as well as our doctor.

Every Thursday, my husband, Bob, brought a friend home from the office to share dinner with us. One night he commented on the amazing desserts I served each week. I had a cake decorating class in my home on Thursday mornings, and each week for dinner I served a beautifully decorated cake. When he complimented me, I realized that every Thursday I was feeding my son dessert covered with artificial flavoring and coloring. It wasn't Robbie's school that was making him sick every weekend . . . it was me!

As I think over those years, I realize how good God was to us in providing a physician specially trained in the United States to be Robbie's doctor. I was so grateful to determine what was triggering Robbie's attacks. Most of all, in spite of all the difficulties caused by Robbie's asthma, I am thankful for the many hours I spent with him, sitting by his bed and holding his hand as he struggled to breathe. We became very close because of those difficult nights. God was faithful and met our every need.

Sometimes it takes a little longer than it should for us to realize how good God is to us. I'm so glad it is never too late to be thankful and to express our gratitude to our wonderful and patient God.

Father, thank You for Your patience with me. Sometimes it takes me a long time to realize how You have blessed my life and protected me. Thank You for Your faithfulness in caring for me and for my family. I love You and want to be aware of Your presence in my life daily.

Journal: Think about a situation in the past when you found it difficult to be thankful. Has your perspective changed? How?

GIVING THANKS OR FEELING THANKFUL?
by David Self

God's Word commands us to "give thanks" about 135 times. How is *giving thanks* different from *feeling thankful*? Giving thanks is an action that implies specificity; feeling thankful is passive and deals in generalities. Giving thanks recognizes the One who is the source of our blessings; feeling thankful may not even acknowledge our Source. Giving thanks ultimately gives glory to God; feeling thankful only makes us feel good about ourselves.

What about the "all circumstances" part of this week's verse? How literally do we take that? Elisabeth Elliot said, "It is always possible to be thankful for what is given rather than to complain about what is not given. One or the other becomes a habit of life." Even in bad circumstances, we can find reasons to give thanks.

My wife, Bonnie, and I were having a difficult Christmas season due to her mother's health. Rose had rather suddenly developed double vision and was experiencing painful headaches. She had visited multiple doctors and undergone many tests.

While my wife and I were traveling north on I-45 to see my side of the family for Christmas, her cell phone chirped. "This is the doctor's nurse. Your mother's MRI has revealed a spot in her brain that may be malignant. Can we schedule an appointment with the doctor after Christmas to discuss treatment options?" Just like that, the axis of our world seemed to pivot; everything seemed to change.

We exited the interstate and pulled into a vacant lot, with a thousand questions on our minds. *What does this mean? Should we cancel our trip? Is this the right time, just before Christmas, to tell Rose, who is 80 years old?* Feeling terribly alone and discouraged, we held hands and began to pray. Increasingly, our prayers turned to thanks. We thanked God for His love, His power and His care for His children. We admitted our ignorance and lack of direction, but thanked Him for His wisdom and knowledge. We thanked God that, even though we felt out of control, He was in perfect control. Finally, we thanked Him in advance for peace.

After we prayed, I felt that Bonnie should call the doctor for some clarification. I called my brother, a physician. Both doctors offered solid advice and counseled us not to assume the worst. As the diagnosis developed over the next weeks, we found that Rose had a benign cyst, unconnected to her other symptoms. The double vision and headaches required a surgical repair of an eye muscle, which was very successful.

While not everyone's crisis has such a happy ending, every believer can still "give thanks in every circumstance." The very act of giving thanks directs our attention from our helpless position on Earth to God's limitless resources in heaven.

Dear Heavenly Father, I give thanks to You for Your indescribable gift (see 2 Corinthians 9:15), Your inalterable victory (see 1 Corinthians 15:57), Your incomparable inheritance (see Colossians 1:12), and Your inconceivable power (see Matthew 28:18). You are my Source and the One due all praise.

Journal: Have you given thanks today? Make it an "everyday, every circumstance" habit. Make a list of things you can be thankful for today and every day.

THANKFUL IN CHRIST JESUS
by Karrie Smyth

Day
7

My First Place 4 Health journey began because Carole Lewis was faithful to obey God's command in this week's key verse. Carole's daughter Shari was killed in a tragic accident on Thanksgiving Day 2001. Just a few short months later, I heard Carole share of the Lord's amazing faithfulness to her during this time of great loss. She expressed how thankful she was that the Lord had awakened her early that Thanksgiving morning to speak tenderly through His Word. I was amazed at the fact that Carole could give thanks in such horrible circumstances. I wanted a relationship with the Lord like that.

Sometimes I think we don't put enough emphasis on the words "in Christ Jesus" in this verse. It was because of her deep abiding relationship in Christ that Carole could give thanks in her grief. It was God's will for her and it is God's will for us. My life is forever changed as a result.

At one time or another, we all face circumstances when being thankful is a choice. The enemy tells us that we have nothing to be thankful for. Our minds focus on all the reasons that we have to be discouraged. That is when we need to draw ever closer to God and find all we need in Christ Jesus.

Allow Him to wake you in the mornings. Sit with Him and allow Him to speak to you through His Word. He wants to transform you in the midst of those circumstances by the renewing of your mind. He will never leave you or forsake you. He is the Friend that sticks closer than a brother. He will meet all your needs according to His glorious riches in Christ Jesus.

Are you facing tough circumstances this holiday season? Does giving thanks seem impossible? God knows everything you are going through and how you feel. He will never command you to do something that He will not empower you to do. Begin thanking Him that you do not have to face your problems alone. Make a list of the promises He's given you in His Word and thank Him for them one by one. Keep the list in a thankfulness journal or somewhere handy so that you can remind yourself often.

"Give thanks in all circumstances, for this is God's will for you in Christ Jesus." There are people around you who are yearning for what makes that kind of thankfulness possible. You may never know the impact your obedience will have. For Carole's, I am forever thankful!

Lord, thank You that whatever You command us to do, You enable us to do. Help me to choose to be thankful in You today.

Journal: Ask the Lord to open your eyes and heart to see how He is at work even in the worst of your circumstances. Write down your prayer, and as you begin to see His hand in your situation, don't forget to thank Him!

Group Prayer Requests

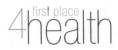

Today's Date: _____

Name	Request

Results

_____

_____

_____

_____

_____

goodness
and love

SCRIPTURE MEMORY VERSE
*Give thanks to the Lord, for He is good;
His love endures forever.*
1 CHRONICLES 16:34

FORGIVENESS AND THANKFULNESS

by Carole Lewis

Day
1

Last week when I opened the mailbox to retrieve our mail, I saw a letter with a return address from the Texas Department of Pardons and Parole. With the anniversary of our daughter Shari's death approaching, I knew, without opening the envelope, that this was the letter letting our family know the time was approaching for a possible parole for the girl that hit our daughter on Thanksgiving 2001.

Lisa Marie DeLeon was driving drunk that fateful night when her car left the road and came down the sidewalk where our daughter Shari stood behind the family car. As I read the letter, my memory bank pulled up that horrible day when Lisa Marie was sentenced to prison in June 2002. She had pled guilty to vehicular homicide and had received a mandatory 12-year prison term. The sentence dictated that Lisa Marie must serve 6 years of that sentence before becoming eligible for parole.

As the memory surfaced, it was not what I expected. Instead of reliving the ordeal of making our victim statements or replaying Lisa

Marie saying how sorry she was to have caused Shari's death, my mind fastened on the moments when we were leaving the courtroom. My son-in-law, Jeff, our three granddaughters and Jeff's parents and siblings exited to the left side of the courtroom while Johnny and I exited to the right.

The next thing I saw was my husband stooping down to hug the weeping mother of 18-year-old Lisa Marie. My husband has the gift of mercy, and he was able to put himself in that mother's place, watching her daughter being led away to prison. I was overcome with love for my Johnny as he demonstrated God-like character in the middle of a devastating time.

As I reflect on why that memory was the first one to come to mind, I am struck by the fact that we all have sinned. There is no degree of sin with God; sin is sin. All of us have sinned and all of us have been sinned against—but forgiveness and thankfulness are the keys that allow the Holy Spirit to transform bad memories into times of learning great spiritual truths.

As Johnny and I read the letter from the Parole Board, we both had the same feeling: We would leave Lisa Marie's parole in the hands of our loving Father. I have sent Lisa Marie a Bible and prayed for her salvation many times in these last six years. I know that God loves her as much as He loves us and we want His perfect will played out in her life and in the life of her family.

Dear Lord, You are good and Your love endures forever.
Because of this, I can give thanks in every circumstance of life.
I pray that Your love for me and for those who have hurt me
will bring great glory to Your name.

Journal: This Thanksgiving season, is there someone God wants you to forgive? Is there someone or some circumstance in your life that you can begin praying about?

Day
2

GREAT AND GOOD
by Jim Clayton

My wife and I have eight precious grandchildren between the ages of 2 and 9. When we are all together, it is so much fun to hear them debate over who is going to say the blessing before our meal. This is especially true when we have our family together for Thanksgiving.

The four older grandchildren are beginning to learn to say words of thanksgiving from their own hearts, but I must confess that it's the four younger ones I enjoy most, even though we know what the words of the blessing will be. Holding hands in a large circle, one of them begins, "God is great! God is good! Let us thank Him for our food. By His hand we all are fed. Thank You, God, for daily bread. Amen!" It's the same every time and the words have not changed, at least not in the last 50 years; it is the same blessing I first learned when I was their age.

And the theology could not be more accurate.

The words of that blessing echo what the writer of Chronicles says in this week's key verse. God is indeed *great* and *good*. I mean, that's who He is. It is His very nature. He could not be anything else. His grace, love, mercy, patience and even His righteous judgments are characterized by who He is . . . and who is He? He is *great* and *good*. I don't know that our two-year-old granddaughter yet recognizes just how awesome God is, but she does acknowledge that He is *great* and *good*. It is from Him that our bountiful food originates. It is by His hand that we are fed. And it is because of Him that we can express our gratitude for what He provides this day.

Our family has another Thanksgiving tradition. With the aroma of food filling the dining room and everyone anxious to enjoy the meal, we again join hands and everyone tells at least one thing he or she is thankful for. With the kids, these things are likely to be "my kitty cat," "my puppy," "my baby doll" or "my video games." As the older age group begins to respond, they may be "my health," "my spouse," "my job" or "my family." Inevitably, someone says, "I am thankful for *Jesus*, because without Him, all of this would be so meaningless, so empty."

Let me encourage you during this Thanksgiving season to quietly and simply *give thanks to the Lord, for He* is *good; His love* does *endure forever*. Our grandchildren often say it best because they don't have to impress us with their words: "Papaw, God is *awesome*, isn't He?"

He is indeed, Jacob! He is indeed!

Father, help me today to be truly thankful
and to express my thanksgiving to You with my life
as well as with my lips. Help me to know that I am
only blessed because of Your mercy and grace.

Journal: In what ways can you express your thanksgiving to a loving God today? How can you *show* Him, as well as *tell* Him of your thanksgiving?

PRAISE THE LORD, O MY SOUL
by Elizabeth Crews

Day
3

When I first came to know Jesus Christ as my Savior and Lord, God's enduring love was a concept I could not even begin to fathom! I was the product of a home where love was conditional. If I was polite and agreeable, if I obediently did all I was asked to do without complaining—if I cleaned my plate at mealtime, got good grades in school and made no demands on my parents—then I was loved. But the moment I showed any sign of weakness or rebellion, the "love" quickly went away, sometimes for days.

As a result, I developed a lifestyle of pleasing others at the expense of self. The words "No" and "I'm not able to do that" were just not part of my vocabulary—and as a result, I was dying inside. Hopes and dreams gave way to what we now call "people-pleasing," letting others control my destiny rather than being responsive to God's will. Hearing that God's love in Christ Jesus was unconditional and enduring was not a concept I could wrap my mind and heart around, much less put into practice.

I clearly remember the day I asked God to prove Himself worthy of my trust. I was meditating on the words of Psalm 103:1-5. I knew God as the one who forgave all my sins and healed all my diseases. I knew that He had redeemed my life from the pit and put my feet on solid ground. I had experienced being crowned with love and compassion.

However, when it came to renewing my strength and satisfying my desires with good things, I was not at all convinced God could or would do those things for me, not after the mess I had made of my life and the high cost I had paid for pleasing others rather than pleasing Him! Even now, as I write these words, I wonder where I found the courage to be so bold as to ask God to prove Himself to be my Renewing Provider, that He would renew my strength and satisfy my desires with good things. Such brave words are not usually part of the humble stance I take in God's presence.

To my surprise, not only did God hear my words, He answered my prayer. And He did so in a very interesting way. Rather than scolding me for my humble boldness or withdrawing His love because I had made a request of Him, He brought me to First Place 4 Health.

As I have been faithful to practice the First Place 4 Health program, God has proven Himself faithful beyond my wildest imaginings. My physical health is being restored, my emotions have stabilized, my thoughts have become concise and clear—and my spirit has begun to soar like an eagle! As for satisfying my desires with good things, He has satisfied my deep longing for unconditional acceptance by giving me His enduring love. As a matter of fact, when I have been most unlovable, God has loved me the most. While I was still a sinner, Christ died for me.

Thank You, Gracious God, for all Your benefits. You have forgiven my sins and healed my diseases. You have redeemed my life from the pit and set my feet on solid ground. You have crowned me with love and compassion, and You have renewed my strength. Today my spirit can soar because You have satisfied my desire for enduring love and unconditional acceptance in Jesus Christ my Lord.

Journal: Read the words of Psalm 103:1-5 and talk to God about how you have experienced His many benefits through participation in First Place 4 Health.

GIVING OF OUR BEST
by Bev Schwind

The Spanish-speaking congregation used the same church building as we did for their services, and many of us English-speakers began to learn some of the worship songs in Spanish. Most of the people in the congregation were poor and some were in the U.S. on their own, working to make enough money to bring their family here.

After their service each Sunday afternoon, a group of us prepared dinner for them. It was always fun to see them come through the doors and see the smiles on their faces as they looked at the buffet of home-cooked food. Our pastor suggested that we prepare a traditional Thanksgiving meal and also honor the children who had birthdays that month. We were excited about decorating for the event, even purchasing a piñata for the children, incorporating traditions from both cultures.

The dining room was also prepared. We put tablecloths on the tables, plus candles and appropriate decorations. The room looked beautiful. We gathered outside as the children took turns trying to break the piñata and get the goodies that were inside, waiting in anticipation for the congregation to come through the doors.

I was stunned when one particular woman came into the room, wearing a dress that I had always loved. I had been led to give away the dress when I was told of a dire situation. In the past it had been easy for me to give away things I did not like, but it was incredible to see a favorite garment on a woman who looked as if it had been designed for her. When I saw that dress, I had a hard time not weeping as I thanked God for leading me to give away a favorite item. I could tell she liked the dress too, and I secretly smiled to myself and thanked God for the lesson.

We all agreed Thanksgiving was a good idea. It did not matter that there was a language difference in our fellowship; we felt the same love of the Father. Together, sometimes using an interpreter, we exchanged stories. Thanksgiving was giving thanks to the Lord for His goodness and mercy that endure forever.

> *Holy Lord, we are thankful that Jesus is a gift of salvation for all people. Help us to eagerly share our earthly possessions, but most of all lead us to share Your gospel with others. Thank You that Your love endures forever.*

Journal: This holiday season is a good time to tell others why this is a *holy* season. What can you give to God and to others that is your very best?

SING PRAISE
by Erin DuBroc

I will never forget the summer of 2003. My dad and I were making a long and winding roadtrip to Durham, North Carolina, where I was completing a summer internship at Duke University. Instead of taking the most direct route from Houston, we took the scenic route and stopped at every state line to take pictures, basking in the fun of it all. I always had a great relationship with my dad, but that trip added to its sweetness. We talked, laughed and sang aloud to my new James Taylor *Greatest Hits* album ("Carolina in My Mind" played just as we crossed the Carolina state line). God knew exactly what I needed. It was a precious few days. In spite of the prostate cancer diagnosis Dad had received just months prior, the world seemed perfect. He was asymptomatic and not even undergoing serious treatment. It all seemed under control.

The summer flew by. When it was time to make the drive home, I learned that Dad would not be flying in to make the trip back with me. Dad flew in my dear friend Nikki to drive home with me, and again . . . God knew what He was doing. The trip was full of more sing-a-longs and laughter. I wasn't given any specific reasons for Dad's absence, but deep down I began to suspect that his health had taken a downturn.

When I arrived home, the truth was obvious. My dad was pale and tired, and though he mustered up enough strength to smile and assure me that everything was fine, I knew everything wasn't. I was scheduled to fly only two weeks later to Italy for a semester abroad. When I realized the truth of my father's condition I was opposed to the trip, but my parents were determined that I should go. Reluctantly, I boarded a plane in late August. Two weeks later, I got the dreaded phone call: Dad had passed away from complications during chemo treatment.

For the past few years, I've been learning how to grieve, accept, move forward and everything else that comes with bereavement. There is no instruction manual for the process, but God has walked with me every step of the way—just as He did by making it possible for Dad and me to have those cherished few days on the road together.

It was several months after my dad's death until I could listen to "Fire and Rain" by James Taylor, our favorite song on the road trip. When I did, I heard God whisper, "I am watching over you, Erin. I'm holding you up today and I will be here again tomorrow. I know you're hurting and tired, but trust Me to help you through this . . . I will." He has, and I can't help but sing His praise. He is so good and His love endures forever.

Precious God, thank You for Your goodness and enduring love.
Tune our ears to hear the songs You sing over us (see Zephaniah 3:17),
full of healing words and comforting melodies, and help us to sing
praise in all circumstances, for we know You are above all things.

Journal: Sing praise to God today! In your heart, on the pages of your journal, through the words of your mouth . . . sing praise!

SHOWER OF BLESSINGS
by Barbara Lukies

Day
6

One of the ladies in our First Place 4 Health group lost everything in a house fire. The only thing she had left were her family (who made it out alive) and the clothes on her back. Despite these tragic circumstances, she continued to attend First Place 4 Health. Her family had been through so much pain already and it seemed as if a big commitment was the last thing she needed in her life . . . but as the weeks and months went on, I saw God do a miraculous work in her life.

She picked up the pieces and began to build a fresh life. People in our group and others in our community donated finances for a new, fully furnished house—debt free. The family was given brand-new clothes, and the lady commented to me that they had never had new things before.

As God poured out His love and blessings upon her and her family, she began to change. When I first met this lady, she had been a housebound person who was not comfortable going outside, into the public eye. She was very overweight and many times very discouraged, ready to give up on her weight loss. Yet as she experienced God's goodness, she continued to join the group discussions and her mindset was slowly changed. Things of the past began to heal. Her weight has started to drop.

She has also begun to give back to others by providing childcare and creating beautiful wood-lathed pens. Her pen-making has won awards; she has been asked to display her creations in art galleries. She has learned how to cook healthy meals and how to fit exercise into her day by walking other people's children to school. She is no longer housebound and has a newfound confidence.

As the goodness and enduring love of the Lord has shone through her circumstances, she has learned to give thanks.

Lord, we thank You for the privilege of walking alongside others
in their journey and seeing how Your love transforms lives.
We give You thanks, for You are good! Your love does endure forever.

Journal: Is there someone close to you who has experienced the goodness and love of the Lord raining down upon them during the past year? Write how God has blessed them, and thank Him for His enduring love.

DELIGHTFUL SURPRISES
by Dee Matthews

Day

7

At the end of last spring's First Place 4 Health session, we were all looking forward to some time away from the weekly preparations for our group meetings. As we shared our excitement, I was asked if I planned to help with the six-week summer session. I'm afraid that I was a little emphatic in stating that I was not interested . . . period!

Well, I'm not sure exactly how it happened, but somehow I went from not being interested to coordinating all six meetings that summer. One minute I was strongly saying that I would not do it, and the next minute I was agreeing to lead the whole summer session!

I will always be so glad that I made that decision. I am thankful that God knows the plans He has for me (see Jeremiah 29:11) and that His thoughts are not my thoughts (see Isaiah 55:8). I thought I did not want to work with First Place 4 Health in the summer, but God had something special in store for me. The summer session turned out to be a great experience in my life.

The ladies who attended the summer session were fantastic. We had a great time, and I learned so much from each of them. Two ladies from the spring session volunteered to help me, and they were so encouraging. I was able to spend some very special time with them. How I love them both!

The best part of the session was one of our memory verses. Psalm 143:8 says, "Let the morning bring me word of your unfailing love, for I have put my trust in you. Show me the way I should go, for to you I lift up my soul." What a wonderful promise from His Word! Every night as I turn off the light to go to sleep, I say that verse to the Lord. I awake in the morning filled with confidence that God has a special word just for me and that He will guide me as I go through the day, as I humbly lift up my soul to Him. What a comfort that verse is for me still.

How very thankful I am that I decided to be involved in the summer session. Truly His love endures forever, and He reassures us of His unfailing love daily.

Father, I love the way You surprise me with special blessings,
even when I fail to see the opportunities that You bring into
my life. O Father, I want to be available to You.

Journal: How has God blessed you in the last year with an opportunity to serve and glorify Him? Express your gratitude for His invitation to live with purpose each day.

Group Prayer Requests

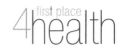

Today's Date: _____

Name	Request

Results

_____

_____

_____

_____

_____

Week Three

great
joy

SCRIPTURE MEMORY VERSE

*But the angel said to them, "Do not be afraid. I bring you good news
of great joy that will be for all the people. Today in the town of David
a Savior has been born to you; He is Christ the Lord."*
LUKE 2:10-11

Day
1

DO NOT FEAR
by Carole Lewis

Those four little words, "Do not be afraid," spoken to some shepherds
in a field outside of Bethlehem over 2,000 years ago, are still powerful
today. Fear is a paralyzing emotion that makes us ineffective for God's
use on a daily basis. This is why God tells us "Do not fear" so many
times in the Bible.

An acronym for F.E.A.R. is False Evidence Appearing Real. Several
years ago, I had an experience that shows the debilitating power of fear
and confirms the truth of that acronym. My husband, Johnny, was in
the middle of a round of chemo when he began to have serious bouts
of pain in his stomach. One of these bouts happened at two o'clock in
the morning. I was awakened by Johnny tapping me on the shoulder,
saying, "We need to go to the hospital." I knew he must be in terrible
pain, so I jumped up, dressed and drove him to the hospital as quickly
as possible.

At the hospital, Johnny was diagnosed with acute pancreatitis. The doctors said that he would need to stay in the hospital until he improved enough to have his gallbladder removed. Fear began to creep into my heart; I just knew that Johnny's cancer was the culprit and that his cancer had now spread to his gallbladder. As the fear grew, I could envision the doctor finding cancer everywhere when he operated. My mind even jumped ahead to the hospital bed that we would put in our bedroom when Johnny returned home.

Did I voice my fears to family, coworkers or friends? Of course not; I thought I needed to bear up and get ready for the worst. Instead of asking for support and encouragement, I fed my fear with food from the cafeteria and the gift shop at the hospital. I ate pie and candy bars every time I was away from Johnny's room. In some weird way, I believed that I was helping the situation.

When the day of surgery finally came, the doctor came out to say that Johnny's gallbladder was gone and everything else looked good. Today, two-and-a-half years later, everything still looks good. Johnny still has stage-4 prostate cancer, but his latest bone and CAT scans show no cancer growth at all.

All I had to show for my fear was internal stress and external weight gain. I have found it to be true that most of the time, the things we worry about never happen.

Dear Lord, help me when I
am afraid to trust in You, for You,
Lord, have never forsaken
those who seek You.

Journal: Talk to God about your fears. Ask Him to help you trust Him enough to let go of your fears and trust them to His loving hands.

GOOD TIDINGS OF GREAT JOY
June Chapko

I do not like change! I find comfort in the familiar and satisfaction in succeeding at what I've done over a long period of time. When I began driving many years ago, I took a familiar route to visit a friend, never detouring. I knew how long it took me to get there and which streets to turn on. It took me five years to discover a quicker way because I feared getting lost. After my friend showed me the new way to go by riding with me, I was forever grateful to her for helping me overcome my fear of change.

When I read this week's key verse, I can relate to the fear the shepherds must have felt upon hearing the news of the birth of a Savior who would deliver them. The angels broke into their daily routine of shepherding, and the whole landscape was bathed in bright light from the glory of the Lord. Up to this point, the shepherds had probably been quite content doing what they do best as they always had, but they suddenly were confronted with a frightening situation. They may have thought, *What will happen now?* But the angel reassured them, "Do not be afraid. I bring you good news." Then an entire army of angels came, praising God. Soon the shepherds joined in and were excited and joyful.

Christmas is a joyous celebration of the birth of our Savior. We experience many opportunities to praise God for His Son during the holidays at parties, pageants and prayer gatherings. With all these events, however, comes the fear of getting off track and losing momentum with our eating and exercise. We may be so fearful that we decline to attend functions at church or enjoy the company of Christian friends. We don't want to change our pattern. God's angels would tell us, "Do not be afraid. I bring you good news." God will send an army of angels to show us a different route to take throughout the holidays so that we can avoid getting lost or having our success wrecked because of wrong holiday food choices.

Our Savior wants us to enjoy the holidays with friends and celebrate His birth. He can help us maintain our weight-loss success during this joyous time of year. We only need to ask Him to go along with us to each event to guide our choices.

Have you asked Jesus to ride with you today?

Lord, I rejoice in celebrating Your birth with family and friends. Help me to focus on You and the love You have given to those You have chosen. I pray that I'll remember to give to others the knowledge of that love.

Journal: List upcoming holiday events on your calendar and ask Jesus to attend them with you. List some ways you can prepare ahead of time to stay on track with your eating plan. Ask yourself, *What would I focus on if Jesus were standing next to me at each event? Would I gorge on the food or be filled with celebrating His presence?*

CHRISTMAS WARMTH THROUGH THE LONG WINTER
by Becky Sims

I love Christmas. It is a beautiful time of year, full of lights, music, and visits with family and friends. It is the season of traditions. We try to be more charitable, thinking of others in need. We have gratitude and share a special kinship with others that is not as prevalent at any other time of year. The Spirit of Christ is alive in our hearts.

I have a special attachment to this holiday because I gave birth to my firstborn son on Christmas. I can relate to how special a new baby is to his mother, how precious and loved. He is so small and vulnerable, yet so full of hope and promise.

Sometimes, we get so caught up in the excitement of this season that we forget Jesus grew up to be a man. "Jesus grew in wisdom and stature, and in favor with God and men" (Luke 2:52). Jesus came into the world to teach us how to live our earthly lives. He followed God's will, accomplishing what He was sent to do. He was willing to die on the cross for our sins.

How precious we are to God because He loved us first! How wonderful to know that we will be in eternity with Him! But we do not have to wait until we go to heaven to be close to Him. "God is our refuge and strength, an ever-present help in trouble" (Psalm 46:1). "My help comes from the LORD, the Maker of heaven and earth" (Psalm 121:2). He is available to us through His Word and through prayer at any time.

Yes, "Jesus is the reason for the season." He is worth so much more than any present we might find wrapped beneath our tree. But His purpose should be remembered all year long. We need to remember that even as this holiday season passes and the long winter sets in, the joyful meaning endures forever through our Savior's birth, death and resurrection. We must keep Christ in our hearts and feel the joy that is available even in the winters of our lives. Though we may not be happy with our current circumstances, we can be joyful. We have been given grace and peace through the knowledge of His promise: "For God so loved the world that he gave his only begotten Son, that whoever believes in him shall not perish but have eternal life" (John 3:16). We need not be afraid. Our Lord gave us everlasting life through His beautiful baby boy.

Lord, thank You for giving me the best gift of all—Your Son, my Savior.
Help me to remember the true meaning of Christmas every day of the year.

Journal: Take a few minutes to reflect on the gifts God has already given to you. Keep this list close at hand for the next few months, to warm your heart through the winter.

Day 4

SHARING PEACE
by Barb Lee

In my relationship with my Savior, I never get bored. He throws curves better than any pitcher on Earth.

His pitch to me this year was the gift of peace during the normally hectic season. Not just joy, but peace—calm, lack of hurry. With cards out and decorating finished right after Thanksgiving, I couldn't even scare up worry or last-minute panic. With a grateful heart I asked, *Why, Lord?*

His answer seemed to be, *Find those in need and share the gift that I have given you.* As I walked away from a friend's house after quickly dropping off a present, I understood His answer. Even though my friend *liked* the present, she needed the gift of my unhurried time and attention.

This year, I have been able to stand back and observe life without being in the middle of it. I have seen physical pain, loneliness, grief, fatigue, stress, worry, anger, sickness, depression and deep sadness in the lives of friends, family members, coworkers, students, store clerks, salespeople and fellow drivers. And I have been able to share the peace that Christ has given me with many.

I've found that if you have the time to ask a cashier how she's doing and then wait for an answer; to sit with an elderly friend; to listen to a frustrated worker, wife or father; or to help someone who is sick or suffering, you don't have much competition at Christmastime. Everyone else is too busy! What an opportunity to share the love of our Savior, the Prince of Peace, when it is most needed!

Prince of Peace, Your birth was the best news this world ever received! Help me to reflect Your love to others this season with a smile, a kind word, or a listening ear. Remind me that You are the true reason for the season.

Journal: Write a prayer asking the Lord to grant you peace this season so that you may share it with others. Record what you do and the responses you get from others so that you can remember them next year!

CONQUERING FEAR
by Elizabeth Crews

Prior to coming to First Place 4 Health, fear was the emotion that defined my life: fear of failure, fear of scarcity, fear of rejection, fear of inadequacy. The list was endless, but the root cause was always the same: fear of not being enough. In the core of my being, I felt irreparably flawed, helpless and hopeless. Sometimes the fear was tied to specific things that were happening in my life. At other times the fear took the form of free-floating anxiety that seemed to come out of nowhere and resulted in debilitating panic attacks that had devastating physical symptoms: heart palpitations, sweaty hands, shortness of breath. Instead of going from victory to victory, I went from fear to fear, never knowing where or when my archenemy fear would once again rear its ugly head.

What I have now learned is that some of my angst was a chemical reaction to the high-sugar diet I was eating, which, coupled with a chronic lack of exercise, left me vulnerable to emotional mood swings. Like my weight, my emotions were up or they were down, but they were never moderate. Following the Live It plan helped level out both my roller-coaster emotions and my weight fluctuations.

However, not all of my anxiety could be attributed to poor diet and lack of exercise. It has been said that the battleground we fight is primarily in the mind, and for me this was especially true. The negative voices that chattered endlessly in my head were the main cause of my fear. As David declared in Psalm 3:1-2, I had many foes telling me there was no hope for me in God—and most of them were inside my own head! This was obviously a battle to be waged with divine weapons, not the world's psychology!

At the suggestion of my spiritual mentor, I selected a group of Scripture passages that addressed this thing called fear. And as I began to train my eyes to look for passages of Scripture that address the issue of fear, even the Christmas story took on new meaning. I was struck by the angel's words to the shepherds: "Do not be afraid. I bring you good news of great joy!" And as I meditated on the words of Luke 2:10-11, it became obvious that the command "Do not be afraid" was not about overcoming fear in my own strength and power; it was about freedom from fear because Jesus Christ, my Savior, has been born. Because I have confessed Him as Savior and Lord, there is no condemnation. Praise God! I am accepted in His righteousness.

Today when I read the words of the Christmas story, I have special reason for rejoicing. I have been set free from the fear that kept me from being all that God created me to be. I no longer go from fear to fear. I can celebrate victory because Jesus Christ has overcome the world and invites me to allow His power to conquer all my fears, too.

Thank You, Gracious Lord, for sending Your Word to heal me from all my diseases. When I put my trust in Jesus, I will not give in to the fear that keeps me from loving and serving You with all my heart, mind, spirit and strength.

Journal: What fear keeps you from experiencing the joy of Christmas? And, more important, what passage of Scripture can you use to combat that fear?

JUST A SHEPHERD
by Jim Clayton

Day
6

Picture this scene: Somewhere between Jerusalem and Bethlehem (a distance of only five miles), you sit around a campfire on an incredibly beautiful, star-filled night. It is chilly and you are a shepherd, doing what a shepherd does best—shepherding. Nothing like what you are about to experience has ever crossed your mind. After all, you are *just* a shepherd.

Suddenly, the sky is illumined above you with a brightness more brilliant than the noon-day sun. The first words you hear are, "Now, don't be afraid!" *Right*—don't be afraid. Remember, you are *just* a shepherd. Then comes the announcement that will change history forever. An angel speaks, and the words are unmistakable: "I have come with *good news*. Today, just over in Bethlehem, a Savior has been born to you, *just* a shepherd! Now, this *good news* has been placed in your heart, and you will be compelled to share it."

"Don't be afraid." *Okay, but the Messiah has been born, and the news was delivered by an angel to me*—just *a shepherd!*

In August 1993, I was serving as *just* a shepherd in a church in East Tennessee. I was an extremely overweight, out-of-shape shepherd, a high-blood-pressure, short-of-breath shepherd, but I was able to tell my "flock" each Sunday: "Jesus is not only our *Savior*, He also desires to be our *Lord*, our Ruler, our Master." The words were true, but I was a poor example of a shepherd.

Someone introduced me to a life-changing program called First Place 4 Health, a Christ-centered program unlike anything I had heard of before (and I had heard of all of them, believe me). Based on Matthew 6:33, it said that if I would "seek *first* the kingdom of God, and *His* righteousness," then all the other things I needed would be added to me as needed. But I was afraid, really *afraid*. I had tried it all and failed every time. What if I failed again? After all, I was *just* a shepherd.

Then came these very words: "Don't be afraid!" I took that statement and ran with it. By the time Christmas 1993 had arrived, I was almost 40 pounds lighter and walking 3 miles a day. My blood pressure was getting under control and I was no longer afraid. The 40 pounds became 50, then 60, and by the time I had reached "maintenance," I had lost almost 80 pounds! But the best news was that I was no longer afraid, and in the process, I had become a better shepherd!

If you are struggling and dissatisfied with yourself this Christmas season, don't be afraid. Jesus is still Savior, and in His role as Lord, He will bring you where you want to be. And that is still good news!

Father, You have given us "good news" to share in our troubled world.
Help me today, in every area of my life, to tell the Good News of Your Son
and my Savior. Renew my heart where necessary, that I may boldly
proclaim the reason for the coming of the Messiah to a lost world.

Journal: Are you effectively sharing the message of the angels with your world, or are you keeping it to yourself? How can you, during one of the most hectic times of the year, be bold in heralding the Good News?

TWO-DEGREE SHIFTS TOWARD GOOD NEWS
by Judy Marshall

I dearly love good news! Doesn't everybody? Good news takes many forms: a child's birth, the birth of a grandchild, an engagement, a long-awaited promotion, a daughter-in-law accepting God's salvation, a deserved retirement, a disciplined life showing healthy results, observances of spiritual growth in children, and so many more.

A piece of good news I learned last summer was about the small steps we make that result in great changes in our lives. It is rarely a lack of desire to change, but the bigness of the changes that discourages us. We become overwhelmed by the magnitude of all that needs to be changed in us. We desire the end result—the big picture—yet refuse to set small, realistic goals allowing God to reach His intended purpose in us.

In a flight to the moon, a two-degree change would cause the spacecraft to miss its target by over 11,000 miles. Obviously, a minute change in direction can make quite a remarkable difference in the outcome. One-hundred-and-eighty-degree changes in our lives are almost impossible, yet over time, many two-degree shifts in a positive direction move us toward our goal of becoming balanced and healthy—more like Jesus.

What two-degree changes can we make in the four areas of First Place 4 Health that lead to a healthy, balanced life? We can reject one temptation at a time. We can evaluate the reasons we want to eat when we aren't really hungry. We can record our blessings in a journal, increasing the number as we learn to recognize them. These are two-degree emotional changes.

We can begin our exercise plan with a five-minute walk and increase it by a minute each day. We can eat a healthy salad each day. We can drink water before a meal. We can eat before we get too hungry. We can snack on fruits and vegetables. We can sit down at each meal and chew slowly. These are two-degree physical changes.

We can memorize one verse, one word at a time. We can make plans for meals for the family rather than grabbing unhealthy fast food. We can convert a favorite recipe into a healthy First Place 4 Health recipe. These are two-degree mental changes.

We can draw near to God one prayer at a time. We can read and meditate on God's Word for five minutes the first day and increase it by one minute each day. We can listen to praise music in the car or instead of watching TV. We can begin a prayer and praise journal one sentence at a time. We can read one hymn a day. These are two-degree spiritual changes.

When we focus on ourselves instead of God, we sacrifice the eternal on the altar of the immediate. We make selfish choices that are not pleasing to God. The good news is that when our life is total worship and intentional obedience, God can and will bless us. We must allow God to control and balance our daily lives, one small step at a time. He will give us the grace to surrender to His change, for His plan is perfect. News can't get any better than this!

God, thank You for Your love and for the
Good News of salvation. Help me to be bold in making
small steps that shift my course toward You.

Journal: What small two-degree change are you willing to make that will impact your present health journey? Go to www.smallstep.gov for more ideas.

_____

_____

_____

_____

_____

Group Prayer Requests

4 first place
health

Today's Date: _____

Name	Request

Results

_____

_____

_____

_____

_____

Week Four

come
to worship

SCRIPTURE MEMORY VERSE

*After Jesus was born in Bethlehem in Judea, during the time of King Herod,
Magi from the east came to Jerusalem and asked, "Where is the one who
has been born king of the Jews? We saw his star in the east and have
come to worship Him."*
MATTHEW 2:1-2

Day
1

WISE WORSHIP
by Carole Lewis

What does it mean to me personally when I think about those wise men?

They must have made great preparations for the journey. They had a long
way to travel, and wanted to bring their very best gifts to the new King.
They must have thought long and hard about what they would need to
go the distance. Likewise, when I joined First Place 4 Health, I began a
journey that continues even after all these years. Preparation for me
means that the spot where I worship Jesus is always ready with my
Bible, Bible study book, journal and devotional book. I also prepare by
getting enough rest and setting my alarm clock early so that I have
plenty of time for worship.

They took time away from their regular duties to make the journey. It took
time for the magi to make their trip, time away from their work and families to focus on honoring the King. My journey to worship Jesus means
I take care of this body He has given me. In order to do this, I eat healthy

foods and make time for exercise each day. Taking care of my body is an act of worship because I will be able to live longer to better serve Him.

They kept their eyes on the star and didn't take detours. Those wise men had a goal, and they were single-minded in their pursuit of it. True worship occurs when I keep my eyes on Jesus. This means I don't take detours. We believe it took the magi about two years to reach Bethlehem. How many of us who joined First Place 4 Health have taken more years than we care to count because of all the detours we've made along the way? We don't reach the goal because we take our eyes off Jesus.

Dear Lord, I want to worship You this Christmas season. Help me make the preparations, take the time and keep my eyes on You.

Journal: Write something about each of these three areas listed and how you will make this Christmas season a time of true worship.

_____

_____

_____

_____

_____

_____

_____

_____

_____

_____

_____

_____

JOURNEYING TOWARD BETHLEHEM

Day 2

by Elizabeth Crews

Many of our family Christmas traditions have changed since I joined First Place 4 Health—especially those food-related traditions that do not support my year-round commitment to taking care of myself. Gone are the days of containers stuffed with an endless variety of Christmas cookies and pans filled with Grandma's "no fail" fudge—fudge that, true to its name, never failed to add unwanted holiday inches and pounds! Christmas is much simpler now that our family celebrations aren't centered around food. One of the wonderful benefits of First Place 4 Health participation is the freedom to focus on doing the things that nourish my soul rather than clinging to traditions that keep me stuck in destructive patterns that lead to overeating.

But there is one Christmas tradition that has not been eliminated since I joined First Place 4 Health: the nightly lighting of our advent wreath and the intentional placement of the large ceramic nativity set I hand painted and fired over 40 years ago. On the first Sunday of Advent, the stately purple and pink candles are placed in the greenery wreath that sits on a living room table. Next to the wreath is a primitive wooden stable containing just a few animals and an empty manger. The shepherds are placed in the area surrounding the stable. In the northern part of the living room are Mary and Joseph, just beginning the long trip from Nazareth to Bethlehem.

In the eastern part of the room are the magi and their gift-laden camels. Each evening throughout Advent, the appropriate candles on the wreath are lit and a Scripture foretelling the coming of the Messiah is read aloud. Then Mary, Joseph and the magi are moved a symbolic day's journey closer to the stable. Before the candles are snuffed out, I spend some quiet time asking myself if I too have moved one day's journey closer to Jesus as I make my own pilgrimage toward Bethlehem.

Have I taken the next right step in the right direction rather than being swept up in the distractions of the season? Will I have a gift to offer the Christ child this Christmas, the gift of a fit body that honors His coming into the world to give me new life?

By Christmas Eve, Mary and Joseph are in the stable and Baby Jesus is lying in the straw-filled manger. Angels have appeared and the shepherds have come to see exactly what is happening in this humble place. The magi are still in the distance, following the star as they come to worship the newborn King of kings. They will continue their journey until Epiphany. But most important of all, my heart has grown closer to the Lord as I have intentionally made the trip to the manger by keeping Jesus first in all things, instead of being thrown off course by the hustle and bustle that the world calls Christmas.

What time-honored holiday tradition might you need to eliminate this Christmas so that you can worship the King of kings and Lord of lords as He deserves to be worshiped and adored? And most important, what is keeping you from saying no to outdated traditions so that this Christmas you can say yes to God?

Lord God Almighty, You are the King of kings and Lord of lords, the One deserving to be worshiped and adored. This Christmas, help me to put away those family traditions that keep me from keeping You first in my life. You came to give me life. Empower me to honor You in all I say and do.

Journal: Write about a food-related family tradition that you need to eliminate so that you can experience the joy that comes from keeping Christ first in all things.

CHOOSING TO WORSHIP
by Judy Marshall

For Christians, Christmas does not come without worship; the two certainly go together. But can worship come without Christmas? Of course it can, but why should it have to? Let's learn how to worship Christ with our choices each day and turn every day into Christmas, having Christ as our daily focus.

The magi worshiped Christ by bowing before Him and offering Him costly gifts. We can choose to bow before Him to offer, or submit, our daily choices. Each time we make wise, healthy choices, we offer Him our obedience, the submission of our will to His. It's true that gold, frankincense and myrrh were valuable gifts for the Christ child, but God views our intentional and willful obedience as far more valuable than any of those. In 1 Samuel 15:22, God's Word says, "To obey is better than sacrifice."

You may ask, "How can every day become a time of worship?" Wise choices are opportunities to worship God, giving Him the glory and honor He deserves:

Choose to honor God by taking care of your body as you eat and exercise properly. Taking care of His temple acknowledges God as our Maker. "Come, let us bow down in worship, let us kneel before the Lord our Maker" (Psalm 95:6).

Choose to be thankful and give Him praise in what you do. "So whether you eat or drink or whatever you do, do it all for the glory of God" (2 Corinthians 10:31).

Choose to celebrate the holiday season, as well as new life each day, with Christ as the center, rather than focusing on food. This will show your family true worship as you honor God. "But seek first his kingdom and his righteousness, and all these things will be given to you as well" (Matthew 6:33).

Choose to fill your heart and home with Christian music for your soul. "Come, let us sing for joy to the Lord; let us shout aloud to the Rock of our salvation. Let us come before him with thanksgiving and extol him with music and song" (Psalm 95:1-2).

Choose to be Spirit-controlled, disciplined in the healthy choices you make. We must refuse to commit the sin of overeating, or gluttony. This act of obedience brings glory to God. "Do not get drunk on wine, which leads to debauchery [that is, excessive indulgence]. Instead, be filled with the Spirit" (Ephesians 5:18).

Choose to "offer your bodies as living sacrifices, holy and pleasing to God—this is your spiritual act of worship" (Romans 12:1).

The magi of the Christmas story searched for Christ in order to worship Him. Today we don't have to search because we know Christ; and with each simple, intentional act of obedience, we can worship Him.

God, You alone are worthy of my praise and worship.
May I be mindful of my choices today, for each one can honor
You and will become my spiritual act of worship.

Journal: Write out three choices you will make today that will honor God, and then explain how those choices will be an act of worship to Him.

_____

_____

_____

_____

_____

_____

_____

_____

ETERNAL WORSHIP STARTS NOW!
by Betha Jean Cunningham

What do we know about the magi? Some Bible commentaries suggest that they were a caste of wise men specializing in astrology, medicine and natural science. Other scholars call them stargazers, because they definitely studied the stars. They also seem to have had access to prophecies. We usually think of them being three in number because that is the number of gifts they brought to the house where they worshiped our Lord, but we don't really know how many wise men came to Bethlehem. Regardless, the magi and the shepherds were the smartest folks around!

It was no easy trip for the magi. It's likely that they had to travel two years to find the Christ child. Can you imagine spending that much time on a camel? If the wind blew like it is blowing today in West Texas, they also had to fight the dust. Wonder if they had allergies? That would have made the trip much worse! But they did not give up, in spite of the difficulties. They had a mission, and their desire to complete that mission was strong.

Besides introducing others to the Christ child, shouldn't we be studying for signs of Christ's return? That would mean not just reading our Bible, but studying it carefully. It might mean we need to give up some TV time or idle chatter. We might have to watch what is happening around the world and find reliable sources of information to rely on.

Every word we speak, every deed we perform shows how much or how little we are preparing for Christ's return to Earth. Have you spoken to the next-door neighbor or to the person at the next desk at school or in your office? Does your family know Christ in an intimate way? Do you? Are you preparing for the holidays or for celebrating Christ's birthday? Why not plan now to bake a special cake for Jesus' birthday and put enough candles on it to represent those who will be celebrating with you. Between now and Christ's birthday, belt out a few bars of "Happy Birthday, Jesus" as you think about how wonderful it will be to sing praises to Him for eternity. You will enjoy Christmas as much as the magi did when they saw the Christ child, and you and your family will be prepared for the eternal party in heaven!

Abba, Father, as we celebrate Your Son's birthday, may we be mindful to tell others about His birth and sacrifice for all. Help us to look forward in expectation to Your return.

Journal: As you are making your lists and checking them twice, are you putting Christ at the top? Are you leaving time for personal Bible study and prayer? Why or why not?

THE GIFT OF WORSHIP
by Carol Van Atta

"Okay, Mom, I've got my Christmas list almost done. Do you want to see it?" My nine-year-old daughter didn't wait for my answer before pushing the list in front of me.

"Whoa, there! Wait a minute, Missy. Your list looks pretty long this year. Just because it's on the list doesn't mean it will be under the tree." Sighing, I resigned myself to reviewing her extended catalog of neatly organized items. Electronics in one column, clothing in another, other stuff in the "Other Stuff" section. I had to give her credit: She had thought this out and gone to great lengths to make her requests understandable for me.

One obvious thing she had forgotten while preparing her lovely document, however, was the fact that finances were tight and that Christmas is more about giving than getting. But instead of calling her in for one of my infamous lessons on idolatry or a lecture on selfishness, it occurred to me that just maybe I had contributed to this growing greed in my household and in my young daughter's heart. Maybe it was time to read the Christmas story like I was reading it for the first time. Again.

Yes, again. I'm prone to selfishness (not that you are, but maybe you'll relate anyway). I like stuff. Stuff is fun. Stuff gives me a feeling of excitement when I first bring it home. It is only later, when I see people who are hurting, hungry or homeless that I am reminded just how much I have. My family has more stuff than we could possibly need or use in a lifetime. Really.

The Christmas story is all about giving: God giving His only Son to a selfish and self-centered people; a virgin girl giving up her youth and her reputation to give birth to our Savior; a man giving up his wedding night privileges in order to love and protect a woman who was pregnant, but not by him. Christmas is about sacrifice. The magi traveled from afar simply to lay their exotic gifts at the feet of a Baby. How could they not? How can we not? How can I not?

Yet again, I was reminded that my own desire for more and more stuff had set the standard in my household. It was time to lead my children to their knees in worship. For only there would they experience the true gift of Christmas: Jesus.

Dear Heavenly King, forgive me for focusing on the glitz and glamour of Christmas. The stuff that the world offers pales in comparison to Your life-changing light. Instead of seeking more of anything and everything this holiday season, I choose to seek You, for You alone satisfy my soul and delight my heart.

Journal: Do you, like so many others, find yourself caught up in the fanfare of the holiday season? Do you spend more time stretching your budget to give extravagant gifts to impress rather than helping meet the basic needs of those with so little? Maybe it's time to sacrifice and give more wisely. List some ways you might do this.

BRINGING OUR ALL
by Claudia Korff

During the Christmas season, I load my music player with Christmas carols and take off walking! One lap, two laps; on the second lap, my favorite Christmas carol, "O Holy Night," plays. The music and lyrics take me away to that shining evening when Jesus Christ, God's gift of Grace to us, was born. When I hear the lyric, "the weary world rejoices," I think of how many times I have been weary and found hope and strength in God's Word and in prayer, and I am thankful.

Shortly after becoming a member of First Place 4 Health, another Christmas carol began to make an impact on me. Every time I heard "The Little Drummer Boy," God stirred something in my spirit, so I stopped to listen carefully to the words.

I have been struggling with weight loss for many years. I would lose 10 pounds, quit, and then gain more back. In my first meeting of First Place 4 Health, I was assured that if I refused to quit, God would transform my life. And it's true: Every session, God teaches me something that changes my life. When I listened closely to "The Little Drummer Boy," I sensed I was again about to learn something new.

What was it God was trying to tell me? I realized that the little drummer brought all he had to Jesus—his talent, his effort, his love— and did his best for Him. What was the result? He made Jesus smile! In response, my prayer became, "Lord, make me like the little drummer boy. I give You my talents; all that I am. Let me honor You by giving our relationship first place, and strengthen my efforts to build more love for You in my life through practicing the areas of balance in First Place 4 Health, one step at a time. As I determine to take the next healthy step, like the little drummer boy, I want to do my best for You."

My motivation is not just to lose weight. I take the next step in order to worship the King of kings, to make Jesus smile.

Three laps, four laps. Now I find I am smiling back at Him!

*Father, I bow down to worship Your gift to me, Your only begotten Son,
Jesus Christ. I praise You that You first loved me and because You did, I now love
You too. Enable me to do my best for You as You empower me by Your grace.
Let me live each day knowing that my relationship with You is true satisfaction.*

Journal: Worship God by meditating on His love for you. Read Ephesians 3:14-21 and marvel at how wide and long and high and deep is the love of Christ. Write in your journal how much you love Him as well. Share a smile together!

FOLLOWING THE STAR
Day 7

by Elizabeth Crews

"We three kings of Orient are/bearing gifts, we traverse afar." Since childhood, I have been fascinated by the strangers from the East who made a long trek across the desert to pay honor to the newborn King. Yet Scripture is curiously silent about the details of their lives. We are told that they came bringing symbolic, prophetic gifts for the King of the Jews: gold, frankincense and myrrh.

According to tradition, the magi were members of the priestly caste of ancient Persia, a group of wealthy men who devoted themselves to knowledge and wisdom—much like Solomon during the golden era of Israel. Perhaps because biblical information on these wise visitors is so sparse, throughout the ages human imagination has attempted to fill in the blanks. Legend tells us there were three wise men, while Scripture only tells us there was more than one.

Folklore even gives us their names: Balthazar, Gaspar and Melchior. Henry Van Dyke wrote a story about a fourth wise man, Artabar, who was delayed as he traveled to meet the other magi and spent the rest of his life seeking Truth. One Christmas, early in my writing efforts, I wrote my own version of the story of the wise men and gave copies to my friends as gifts. (In reading my story today, I see that my friends' greatest gift to me that Christmas was not telling me just how bad the writing really was!)

But while the Bible is vague on many of the details about the magi, we are given three important truths about these wise men: they were *truth-seekers* who were *on a journey* and *prepared to worship*. Perhaps those three sparse facts are what has peaked the interest of writers, artists and storytellers throughout the ages. For deep in our being, the story of the magi is our story, too. Unlike the priests and teachers of the Law who knew the prophecies regarding the Messiah, the magi were not content with head knowledge. Their intent was to worship the newborn King, to turn their knowledge into wisdom that led to worship.

As a member of First Place 4 Health, that is my challenge as well. It is one thing to pour over books—even the Bible—in search of knowledge, but it is another to put that knowledge into action that results in worshiping God with all my heart, soul, mind and strength. It is one thing to read truth, but it is another to earnestly seek truth and begin the long journey that leads to health and wholeness, which is my spiritual act of worship.

Some will be content to read about Jesus this Christmas. Others will begin the pilgrimage to the manger but get distracted by other things. My goal is to keep my eyes on the prize, to follow the star that shines over Bethlehem so that I can worship the King of kings and Lord of lords. First Place 4 Health is for serious seekers who desire to worship God and live for the One who came to die for them. Does that describe you this Christmas?

Thank You, faithful Father, that You promise to reward those
who earnestly seek You. This Christmas I will keep my eyes on Jesus
and come prepared to worship Him in spirit and in truth.

Journal: Describe your seeking, your journey and your preparedness to worship the newborn King of the Jews.

Group Prayer Requests

first place
4health

Today's Date: _____

Name	Request

Results

_____
_____
_____
_____
_____
_____

be made
new

SCRIPTURE MEMORY VERSE

*You were taught, with regard to your former way of life, to put off your
old self, which is being corrupted by its deceitful desires; to be made new
in the attitudes of your minds; and to put on the new self, created to be
like God in true righteousness and holiness.*
EPHESIANS 4:22-24

Day
1

OUT WITH THE OLD
by Carole Lewis

I read somewhere that it is a good idea to get rid of a piece of clothing
every time we buy a new one. By doing this, the article said, we have to
think about whether or not we really need the new piece of clothing before we buy it.

This week's key verse made me think of that article, because so many
times in life, I try to put on the new clothing of righteousness and holiness before I get rid of my old clothing: deceitful desires and old attitudes and habits.

The New Year is a wonderful time to think about how we can get rid
of the old while attempting new things for Christ. This year, why not:

• Trade your old habit of sleeping an extra 30 minutes for the
new habit of getting up to spend that time with God?

- Trade your old habit of watching too much television for the new habit of spending an hour of that time exercising?

- Trade your old habit of making all the department store sales for the new habit of becoming debt free?

This year, my slogan is going to be, "Out with the old, in with the new."

Dear Lord, this year, I want to get rid of the things that are dragging me down. My desire is to put on righteousness and holiness so that I might look more like You. Will You show me what needs to go and what needs to take its place?

Journal: Make a list with two columns, "Old" and "New." Write down the old things that need to go and the new things that need to replace what you throw out.

Old	New

CHANGING THE CLOTHES OF DECEIT
by Marca MacGregor

The excitement of a brand-new year is such a gift, especially for those living in Christ! Full of potential and opportunity, the start of a new year brings about an atmosphere of cheerful optimism. One can practically feel the anticipation in the air.

The season of awaiting the birth of a child parallels that of a new year in many ways. It is a time of optimistic joy for the changes that an infant brings. However, never have I realized how naturally the deception of self occurs than during and following my pregnancies.

I knew by looking at the scale that the weight I had reached was significantly beyond healthy goals. However, each time I saw my image in the mirror, my deceitful desires fostered a level of denial that surpassed my logic. Though I knew the numbers, I continued to believe that I looked just a little heavier than before pregnancy. I deceived myself into believing that my former physical self was not so different from the lady I saw in the mirror.

I believed the lie that I had barely edged past healthy physical boundaries until several months after each of my babies was born. Each time, it took re-submitting to God's parameters for health through joining First Place 4 Health to begin to realize how far I'd strayed. With the passage of time, by reading God's Word and through seeing the documented truth in pictures of my season of self-deceit, I began to realize how wrong I'd been. During the pregnancies, the "computer" of my mind had literally replaced the reality of my reflection with a mirage. This not only happened throughout one pregnancy, but all three. What pervasive self-deception!

Like a computer virus can alter each productive function of the computer it infects, holding on to old destructive attitudes and deceitful desires keeps us from functioning as God intended. It is in the attitudes of our minds that we become new physically and spiritually under God's instruction. Isn't it wonderful to know that we do not have to rely on our own deceptive natures to lead us in choosing a healthy lifestyle? We have the Holy Spirit, ever-present and continually teaching us how to put off the old self and exchange it for the new.

With each choice, let's allow God to make this entire year new with the knowledge that we *can* do as we're told in Scripture. May we make this year bright by daily putting off the corruption of our former selves and wearing the new likeness of His righteousness and holiness.

Father, please show me daily how I can choose to put off my
deceitful, unhealthy ways. Thank You for the exciting knowledge that
my obedience to You throughout this new year will produce a new me,
formed increasingly of Your righteousness and holiness!

Journal: Which "clothes" of your old self has our King readied you to change? What attitudes of your mind will you allow Him to make new so that your life and your health glorify Him this year?

REVERSING THE DOWN SLIDE
by Barb Lee

Day
3

The last week in December, reality strikes. *Why did I buy all those presents, and what am I going to do with all those that were given to me? Where did that extra roll come from? Can a dozen Christmas cookies really cause that? Why was snow so beautiful before, and now I just want it to go away so that spring can come?*

This morning I woke up, looked in the mirror and determined that I needed a face lift, a tummy tuck, a haircut, an eyebrow wax and a chiropractic adjustment. Then it hit me: Christmas was over and I was in "the down slide," the week between the idealism of Christmas and the hope of the new year. The down slide can bring discouragement with the realization that life over the last year just wasn't what we wanted it to be; that we are not who we want to be; that other people are not as great as we'd hoped they'd be; that winter has just set in.

I have found, though, that being in First Place 4 Health eases the discouragement and ushers in hope and joy for all God is going to accomplish in me in the new year. I can look forward to frosty mornings, wrapped in a blanket and warmed by God's Word as I greet the day. Following the Live It Plan insures that I won't keep that "extra roll" for very long. As I do the Bible study, I think of others who may be discouraged and could use a call or a note from me. Before long, my focus is off myself and on loving God and others.

When you put Christ in first place, the down slide quickly turns into the up side!

Lord, thank You for helping me to form new attitudes with which I can serve You better. Thank You for helping me during this holiday season to remember to put my focus on You rather than on earthly things.

Journal: Write about the changes that you want to see in your life in the new year, changes that will reflect your new self in Christ. Then write a short prayer asking God to help you make those changes.

BETWEEN KNOWLEDGE AND OBEDIENCE
by Elizabeth Crews

Deceitful desires. No two words better describe my relationship with food before First Place 4 Health than these! It has been said that addiction is like a craving for salt when we are dying of thirst, and prior to First Place 4 Health, my disordered relationship with food certainly proved those words true. That is why the process of mental renewal has been such an important part of my efforts toward a more balanced life.

Left to my own corrupted reasoning, I consistently chose the wrong foods in the wrong proportions. I find it interesting that these deceitful desires had nothing whatsoever to do with logical thinking or factual knowledge. Somehow the logic and knowledge that I successfully applied to other areas of my life did not come into play when it came to my food decisions. I certainly knew what to do when it came to healthy eating, but putting that knowledge into practice was a different story. Somewhere between knowledge and obedience, deceitful desires crept in and rendered sound reasoning ineffective. I ate peanut butter, even though I knew it would trigger an out-of-control eating episode. I ate that candy bar for the benefits of the sugar rush, even though I knew a corresponding blood sugar crash would soon follow.

To paraphrase the words of the apostle Paul in Romans 7:19, I ate what I knew was harmful and I did not eat the foods that my logical mind told me were beneficial. Deceitful desire, not prudent thinking, dictated my behavior when it came to food! What I desperately needed was a new attitude in my mind—a new attitude that would replace my deceitful desires.

For me, doing what was right, whether I felt like doing it or not, was the key to overcoming the desires that controlled my food choices. It was truly a matter of surrendering my will, which was corrupted by deceitful desires, to God's will, which was for my ultimate good. I acknowledged that God's thoughts are higher than my thoughts and that His ways would bring health and healing.

At first, obedience felt like deprivation! Like an angry child, my corrupted will cried, "This isn't fair!" But little by little, the stubborn will that opposed God's best for me gave way to renewed thinking. I began to see that abstaining from foods I craved was really for my benefit. To continue to abuse my body with food was the real deprivation.

For me, renewed thinking meant replacing immediate gratification with long-term satisfaction—the satisfaction that comes from doing what pleases God, even when it doesn't feel good in the present moment. Even after five years in First Place 4 Health, this putting off of the old self continues to be a daily decision and a Spirit-inspired process. It begins each morning with surrender, and then it filters down to all the food choices I make during that day. By God's grace I am being transformed, and each calendar day is the start of a new year in First Place 4 Health.

O Lord, how thankful I am that You led me to a program such as
First Place 4 Health. On my own, I would have continued to be ruled by my
deceitful desires. Your grace, and Your grace alone, has given me the inspiration
and motivation to enter into the daily process of transformation.

Journal: Spend some time writing about the deceitful desires that keep you in defeat and despair. Then talk to God about your desire to be rooted and grounded in the truth that will transform your mind as you anticipate the beginning of a new year.

PERMANENT RESOLUTIONS
by Jim Clayton

Believe it or not, there are a few things more exciting about the new year than just seeing the "big ball" drop in Times Square. There is something inherently exciting about the opportunity to begin again. Someone very close to me in our church recently said, "Yesterday is now little more than a memory. Tomorrow may never become reality. What we have is the opportunity of today!"

Sometimes I think I co-authored the phrase "New Year's resolutions," but either consciously or unconsciously, we all make them, don't we? Many of us resolve to become healthier now that a new year has begun. We determine to lose weight, join a health and fitness club, quit smoking or begin a regular exercise program. Some resolve to be less stress-filled in the coming year, planning to rest more, spend more quiet time, start a new hobby or stop going to church business meetings (maybe that's just me). Some resolve to be more "spiritual" in the new year, attending church more regularly, becoming more faithful and active, going on our first-ever mission trip, or something simple like reading the Bible and praying more.

A few weeks pass. February or March arrives, and our resolutions are just memories. What happened? We had such good intentions and such motivation!

Paul gives us the step-by-step formula for keeping those New Year's resolutions. We have to (1) "put off the old self," which is the "self" that got us in this mess to begin with; (2) "be made new in the attitudes of our minds," which means change the way we think and the things we think about; (3) "put on the new self," which means changing our dreams, goals and desires; and (4) "be like God in true righteousness and holiness," which is the key to all of this: becoming God-like in righteousness and holiness.

You know, First Place 4 Health is a lot like New Year's resolutions, except we don't have to wait until December 31 or January 1 to decide that we are going to begin again. I once heard a statement by a person much older and wiser than I: "There is only one reason we put erasers on pencils: because people make mistakes!" The need to keep Jesus first in every area of life is a daily opportunity and challenge. Each morning is a new day to begin again.

Dear Father, thank You for making me over, for changing the way
I think about You and about my world, not just on New Year's Day,
but every day of the year. Thank You for picking me up, dusting me
off and helping me to start over.

Journal: As you formulate your New Year's resolutions, are there any changes you need to make in your life? Are they physical? Mental? Emotional? Spiritual? Write down some of these below. The Holy Spirit will help you today to be recreated in true righteousness and holiness.

NEW THOUGHTS FOR A NEW YEAR

by Diane Bagby

Day
6

So often, when a new year rolls around, we are either excited at the prospect of doing something new or are afraid of making a resolution for fear of not succeeding yet again. This year, we need to challenge ourselves not to make a new plan of action but rather a new plan of thinking. Since we tend to act out of what we believe, we should start with what we believe about ourselves. We need to see ourselves as God sees us.

If you have children, think about how you love them. You may absolutely hate a certain behavior, but that does not change the fact that you love your child. Even more, God loves us in spite of our behavior. When our children misbehave, they have consequences to their actions, but hopefully they know that they are still loved. The same is true of us: We should know that we are loved by the Father, even when we blow it.

If we could believe in ourselves the way God believes in us, it would revolutionize our lives. So how do we begin to do that? First, we need to recognize the negative thoughts we believe about ourselves. This week's key verse reminds us to be made new in the attitudes of our minds and to put on our new self. If we don't stop those thoughts and recognize they are destructive, they just keep coming around again and again. Once we recognize them, we can stop them and take charge of them.

Second, we need to remove the thoughts that don't line up with what God says about us. No one knows us better than the One who created us. Let Scripture paint the picture for you of who you were created to be and begin to remove the thoughts that don't line up. Try overwriting them with the Word of God.

Third, we need to renew our minds (see Romans 12:2). Look in your Bible concordance and find Scripture verses that speak to your situation. If you are feeling fearful, and your fear is paralyzing you or keeping you from doing things you know you should, look up the word "fear" in the back of your Bible. Read all of the verses pertaining to your word. Here's one: "God has not given you a spirit of fear, but of power, love and a sound mind" (2 Timothy 1:7). The next time you feel fearful, renew your mind with that verse or another that speaks to you.

Practice this three-step process: (1) Recognize your issue, (2) remove those thoughts and (3) renew your mind with God's Word. In this way, you can change "the attitudes of your mind and put on the new self, created to be like God in true righteousness and holiness." This year, resolve to get some new thoughts.

Dear Lord, help me to see myself as You see me: covered in the righteousness of Your Son, my Savior, full of purpose and promise. Help me to recognize areas in my life that are inconsistent with the picture Your Word paints. Help me to reject the thoughts that don't pass through the filter of Your Word and to be transformed by renewing my mind according to Your Word.

Journal: This week, take a thought-life inventory. Make a chart and write three columns: "The Good," "The Bad" and "The Ugly." Each time you have a significant thought about yourself or someone else, jot it down in one of those three categories. Then go back and apply the three steps detailed above and begin to renew your mind.

The Good	The Bad	The Ugly

The Good	The Bad	The Ugly

CREATING A NEW ME
by Martha Rogers

Since joining First Place 4 Health, I no longer make New Year's resolutions. Instead, I set goals for the year. For each area of my life, I set both a long- and a short-term goal. I think of ways I can put off the life of the previous year and put on a new self, and pray about how I can best create a new me in the four areas of my life.

One year, I set the goal of memorizing each and every Scripture memory verse. Up until then, I had trouble remembering complete verses. The Scripture cards helped, but it wasn't until I started listening to the CDs that the words were written on my heart. Since then, I have managed to memorize most of the memory verses we have studied.

Having God's Word hidden in my heart has changed me. One Sunday at church, the pastor mentioned several verses, and I realized I knew them without looking them up. That was exciting, but the best part of memorizing Scripture is having God's Word in my heart when it's time to face a crisis or give help to someone who needs encouragement.

When our grandson Robert was gravely ill for several months after a liver transplant, I needed God's Word. When I sat with him in the hospital and didn't have a Bible with me, I could recall verses that gave me peace and comfort. So many times I cried over him and pleaded with the Lord to heal his body, and each time I knew the Lord listened and would answer my prayers. Even though Robert still has the disease that destroyed his liver, the new organ is disease-free and completely healthy. He is a happy teenager who knows and understands the goodness and mercy of our Lord.

During the 14 years that I have been involved in First Place 4 Health, the promise of this verse has been fulfilled in my life. My attitudes have changed, my habits have changed, and my relationship with the Lord has changed.

*Father God, may the goals we set for ourselves in the
new year bring honor and glory to Your Name. Help us to
put off our old selves and become like You.*

Journal: What changes does God have in store for you this year? List the changes you'd like to see in your life in the coming year.

Group Prayer Requests

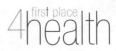

Today's Date: _____

Name	Request

Results

_____

_____

_____

_____

_____

_____

a new heart

SCRIPTURE MEMORY VERSE
I will give you a new heart and put a new spirit in you; I will remove from you your heart of stone and give you a heart of flesh.
EZEKIEL 36:26

HEART TRANSPLANT
by Carole Lewis

Day
1

In this verse, God is talking about giving each of us a heart transplant. He is going to take our old heart and replace it with a new one.

We have a friend who received a heart transplant 10 years ago. He and his wife just celebrated their fiftieth anniversary, and his heart is still working well. Our friend's heart was dying and full of disease when he received his new heart. In the same way, our hearts are dying before we receive Jesus into our lives. A miracle takes place when the Holy Spirit comes to live inside of you and me. He begins to replace our old attitudes and actions with new ones that reflect the new heart living inside us.

Our friend takes many pills each day to keep his body from reject-ing his transplanted heart. In the same way, we care for our new heart by doing those things that keep it from becoming hardened with the world's ideas. The best thing about the new heart God gives us is that our body can never reject it. Jesus says that once He comes to live inside of us, He will never leave us or forsake us.

So what can we do to care for this new heart?

· We can read only what makes our new heart stronger.
· We can watch only what keeps our new heart tender.
· We can listen only to what makes Christ at home in our heart.
· We can eat foods that make our new heart last longer.
· We can exercise to keep our new heart disease free.

Dear Lord, I thank You for this new heart You have given me.
Help me to care for it each day so that I may serve You
in a new way this year.

Journal: Write about ways you can care for your new heart this year.

_____

_____

_____

_____

_____

_____

_____

_____

_____

_____

_____

_____

_____

HEALTHY HEART FOR OTHERS
by Barbara Lukies

My pulmonary valve was opened up this year through surgery. More oxygen was allowed to circulate throughout my body and I entered the new year with a new lease on life. However, my literal "new heart" was just one more step in a process that I began five years ago.

Since joining First Place 4 Health, I've begun to get my eating habits under control, including eating low-fat, low-sugar and low-salt foods. I have been delighted to find that these are neither bland nor difficult to prepare, because I can use herbs and natural juices to add flavor. Eating well has given me more energy; I don't feel uncomfortable after a meal anymore, especially at Christmas.

In the past, I can recall feeling so full after the Christmas meal that I thought I might burst. I can still enjoy healthy food in healthy portions and enjoy celebrating holidays without guilt or being overly full. Since I started eating healthy, I am able to exercise and I have more energy to burn.

But even more profound are the spiritual changes that I have experienced. My heart's desire has become to encourage others in their First Place 4 Health journeys, helping them to see the potential God has for each of their lives. Each member has unique opportunities that God has given him or her to become more Christlike. For some members, He opens doors to a new thought process, while others reevaluate what they feed their bodies. Others are released for ministry, while still others learn new ways of relating in relationships with boundaries and trust, letting go of past hurts so that relationships can be restored or renewed.

Each new year brings exciting changes. With my new heart, I can't wait to witness the changes in leaders' and members' lives, as well as my own, when we daily put God in first place.

Lord, grant me a new heart and a new spirit today. Refresh my soul and heart and remove anything that stands in the way. Replace my heart with joy and a willingness to serve You and others that brings You the honor and glory in this coming year.

Journal: Ask God to give you a new heart and a new spirit. He will do it! He will remove the old and replace it with a new heart to serve Him and others.

Day 3 YOU SAY YOU WANT A REVOLUTION?
by Vicki Heath

Don't you love it when kids use words and don't get them quite right, but somehow what they say still works? Every January when my son Michael was growing up, he asked, "Are we going to make any of those New Year's *revolutions*?" What a great question!

Back in 1968, there was a song by the Beatles called "Revolution" that a few of us may recall. It was on the B-side (a long, long time ago music was released on these little round disks called 45 records) of a very popular song called "Hey, Jude." John Lennon wrote it while attending a transcendental meditation camp in India with the Maharishi. Here's how it starts: "You say you want a revolution, well you know we all want to change the world."

What you may have discovered, along with the Beatles, is that we have very limited power on our own to change anything: ourselves, others or the world. But listen to the words of another writer, the apostle Paul, writing to the believers in Corinth: "Now the Lord is the Spirit, and where the Spirit of the Lord is, there is freedom. And we, who with unveiled faces all reflect the Lord's glory, *are being transformed into his likeness* with ever-increasing glory, which comes from the Lord, who is the Spirit" (2 Corinthians 3:17-18, emphasis added). In other words, God can change us!

God has been the source of a huge revolution in my life. When I was a young girl, He changed my old hard heart into a new tender one. He has also revolutionized my way of thinking. I used to think, *I have to be a perfect example in everything I do: in my weight, in my exercise, in my eating habits, in my personal devotion life, in raising my children.* I could go on and on! Whew! That's a lot of pressure, and it scares me to death just thinking about it. My new way of thinking? *Grace abounds, so strive for excellence and not perfection.*

God, through His Son, Jesus Christ, has provided me everything I need for godliness. Second Peter 1:3-4 says, "His divine power has given us everything we need for life and godliness through our knowledge of Him who called us by his own glory and goodness. Through these he has given us his very great and precious promises, so that through them you may participate in the divine nature and escape the corruption of this world caused by evil desires."

That is what I need to focus on: His power, not my perfection. He promises He will do the work in me and cause me to become the example I need to be for this new year. He is changing me daily into the very image of His Son, Jesus Christ. His living in me is a source of revolutionary power that can directly impact my personal behaviors and my world!

You say you want a revolution? Let God make heart changes in you; then He will use you to *lead* the revolution!

Dear God, this new year I submit my heart to You for Your
continual renewal. I ask that You help me with the changes I need to
make, inside and out, and help me to pass on those changes to the
world around me and have an impact for Your kingdom.

Journal: Are you willing to receive the changes God has in store for you this new year? Are you willing to have a heart change toward those things that have caused you heartache this past year?

STONE INTO FLESH
by Martha Rogers

Day
4

This week's key verse didn't mean a great deal to me when I memorized it several years ago. However, the meaning became crystal clear one January just after New Year's Day. Just before Christmas, my mother called to tell me my brother had again been arrested on drug and sexual abuse charges. His name and picture were all over the papers.

As far as I was concerned, my brother died when he went to prison the second time. I wanted nothing to do with him. That particular Christmas, I had a son getting married and no time to worry about a brother or what happened to him. All I worried about was anyone finding a connection between the man arrested and me.

When Mother called again in January, she told me that Johnny had become a Christian in jail. Her pastor had gone to visit and led my brother to Christ. I couldn't believe it—and didn't *want* to believe it. As I prayed that morning, I didn't feel the peace I usually felt and my prayers seemed to fall flat. I went to school and talked with the chaplain, who handed me a Bible opened to a verse in Matthew. As I read about forgiveness and God's forgiveness, I knew what I had to do. In the chaplain's office, I prayed for God to forgive me of my attitude toward my brother and to soften my heart. If God had forgiven my brother, I could do no less.

I wrote a letter to Johnny and asked him to forgive me for not forgiving him. We had a sweet reunion through our letters, and I realized that God truly had forgiven him. What a wonderful way to start a new year, with a new relationship with my brother! We are now closer than we ever were, even though he is still in prison. He is a child of God and will serve out his punishment knowing that.

When this verse came up in First Place 4 Health, the true meaning of it washed over me. But later, God took my heart of stone and gave me a heart of flesh that learned to forgive and love my prodigal brother.

Thank You, Father, for forgiving my sins. May I have a heart of flesh and love those who have hurt me.

Journal: Do you have a "heart of stone" against someone who has hurt or wronged you? Pray for that person and ask God to give you a "heart of flesh."

MELTING A HARD HEART
by Karrie Smyth

Day 5

I love the promise in the words of this week's key verse! No doubt you, like me, have developed a stony heart at one time or another. We get bumped and bruised by the world around us and we allow ourselves to become hardened in a vain attempt to protect ourselves.

The Lord used this verse to speak hope into a specific season of hardness in my heart. That He would give me a new heart and put a new spirit in me—how amazing! That He would remove from me my heart of stone and give me a heart of flesh, one that is free to love—how incredible! He has taken me back to these words many times. They don't just refer to a one-time work that the Lord wants to do for us; they are words of life for us each and every day.

Ezekiel 36 is full of wise teaching and rich with promise. God's people, the Israelites, were being tossed about relentlessly by the world around them. Their testimony to the watching world was anything but victorious; it was tarnished by their actions and their conduct. But God, for the sake of His Name, declared He would bring them back from where they had wandered. He cleansed them from all of their impurities and from the idols that they had worshiped, and He gave them a new heart.

Perhaps your testimony of victory in the First Place 4 Health program has been tarnished by your own actions and conduct. Perhaps you, like me, have served the idol of food and lost your power to overcome. Maybe you have been bumped and bruised by the world around you and your heart has grown hard. The Lord wants to give you a new heart and put a new spirit in you. He wants to remove from you your heart of stone and give you a heart of flesh. Choose today to come to Him and allow Him to restore your victory. The Lord wants to use you to testify to the watching world that He is mighty and sovereign! His

Holy Spirit, who lives within you, will move you to obedience. For His own sake, He will do this!

In this new year, make it your priority to spend quality and quantity time with the Lord each and every day. He wants to cleanse you from the sins of yesterday and heal the bumps and bruises that you receive from the world. Through your commitment to Bible study and reading, Scripture memorization and prayer, He wants to make you victorious and show the world—through you—what He can do!

Lord, I desire for You to put a new heart within me—one that is
free to love as You love. Please fill me anew with Your Holy Spirit.
I surrender my heart to Your process.

Journal: Ask the Lord to reveal to you any areas where you are allowing your heart to grow hard, and choose to trust Him as He gives you a new heart.

HEAVY WITH GRIEF
by Betha Jean Cunningham

My husband of more than 45 years was gone. I was a widow. I had a lot to learn and my heart was heavy. It may not have been as hard as stone, but it felt as heavy. Four months after Ray's death, I was faced with a brand-new year. I don't remember Thanksgiving that year; I do remember Christmas. My children and grandchildren went out of their way to make it a happy occasion. Then it was New Year's, a time for new beginnings, a time for goal-setting, a time for turning over a few new leaves. I spent time with God and in His Word, but there were times when I got up from my private place and didn't remember what I had read. The music was gone. I could not find the words in my heart.

As a member of First Place 4 Health, I had gotten in the habit of not only doing Bible study but also reading the Bible through over the course of a year. The year before, I had read it through while Ray was ill. I had memorized Scripture, and was so glad to have those verses come to mind while he was declining in health. Jeremiah 29:11, "I know the plans I have made for you" and Isaiah 54:5, "For your Maker is your husband" were the two verses that ran through my mind over and over again. I clung to them like a small scared child to a parent. I hurt. I wanted to seek out what God had in store for me, but the grief was often too great to hear Him.

As the new year approached, I knew I had to shake free from the heaviness in my heart and there was only one way: with God's help. I prayed. I read my Bible daily and studied the First Place 4 Health Bible study. I leaned hard on God as my forty-sixth wedding anniversary came the middle of January. A few days afterward, I found myself singing out loud for the first time in so long! I knew as I sang "His Eye Is on the Sparrow" that I was on my way to a newer life. Oh, my heart still yearns for Ray's familiar voice and his slight touch on my cheek as he walked by, but I can tell my God to let Ray know I will see him some-day—after I've spent the first thousand years with my Jesus!

Almighty God, my Maker, thank You for being everything I need! Thank You for taking a heart heavy with grief and filling it with music again.

Journal: Has something weighed your heart down? Are you staying in God's Word and in touch with Him through prayer? Start now by making a list of your burdens.

A NEW SPIRITUAL HEART
by Elizabeth Crews

It is easy to read Ezekiel's words and think about the new spiritual heart God gives us, replacing our resistant and disobedient heart of stone with a soft, pliable heart that is tender toward the Lord and His commandment. However, for those of us in First Place 4 Health, Ezekiel's words have implications in more than just the spiritual realm!

When I first came to the First Place 4 Health program, years of yo-yo dieting and neglecting my health had taken a very high toll on my physical well-being. I was diagnosed with "syndrome X," or metabolic syndrome: hypertension, high cholesterol levels, high triglycerides, impaired glucose tolerance and insulin resistance. Together, these diseases were hardening my arteries and impairing the function of my heart.

Much like a patient in a triage center, my first priority after joining First Place 4 Health was to stabilize my metabolism. Until that happened, permanent weight loss would not be possible. It would have been futile to concentrate on losing weight when so many other facets of my life were out of control! In the beginning, victory for me was not about watching the scales go down. Victory was seeing the blood pressure readings get lower, the cholesterol and triglycerides drop into the normal range and the blood sugar even out. Victory was about being able to walk 30 minutes a day, not about running a marathon! The few pounds I managed to shed during my first three First Place 4 Health sessions were only a bonus!

Patience with the process is perhaps the greatest lesson I have learned in First Place 4 Health: patience and persistence, even when there is no immediate gratification other than sitting before God at the end of the day, knowing I have done all He asked me to do and taking one more small step in the right direction. Yes, day by day, moment by moment, God is giving me a new heart and a new spirit, a new heart and spirit that impact every aspect of my being and make every day the start of a new year in First Place 4 Health.

O Lord God, You are so loving and patient with me.
Help me to be patient with myself and the process
You are using to give me a new heart and a new spirit.
How can I ever properly express my gratitude to You?

Journal: How has God transformed your heart and spirit through the First Place 4 Health program? Be sure to write about all aspects of your being—physical, mental, emotional and spiritual—because God is active in each of the areas of your life.

Group Prayer Requests

4 first place
health

Today's Date: _____

Name	Request

Results

_____

_____

_____

_____

_____

_____

holiday helps

HOLIDAY SURVIVAL TIPS

Maintaining healthy eating habits and an exercise regimen during the holidays can seem like an overwhelming task. Many times, all of our good habits we have worked so hard to develop are thrown out the window as soon as November arrives! Planning ahead for holiday challenges is the key to surviving the holidays with those healthy habits intact. These suggestions will help you experience a healthier holiday season:

Focus and Prioritize

- Find a holiday exercise buddy to walk with you daily or attend an aerobics class together. Make exercise a priority!

- Find healthy holiday recipes that will fit into the Live It Plan and that you will enjoy serving to holiday visitors.

- Focus on friends and family rather than on food. Make a special gift for each person attending your holiday get-together. Take digital group pictures and place a print in a Thanksgiving card for each person to take home with him or her as a keepsake.

Shopping Savvy

- Park far away from the front door of the mall! Walk briskly, get some exercise and save time looking for a parking space.

- Stop in the name of health! Don't even think of stopping for a treat at the food court! Pack some shopping snacks in your bag: yogurt, raisins, an apple, a banana or pretzels. Planning ahead will prove to be a money saver and a calorie cutter.

- Warm up. Before actually making any purchases, take a stroll through the entire mall, then go back to make purchases. This will not only add steps to your shopping day, but also will help you make informed decisions about your purchases.

Healthy Activities

- Start a neighborhood tradition. Invite your neighbors to walk the neighborhood and sing Christmas carols along the way.

- Volunteer to help a young mom by offering to take her young child for a stroller ride.

- Help out at a soup kitchen, or clean out your closets and donate the items to a local charity.

Party Hearty

- Holiday parties can sabotage your healthy eating plan, but with a little planning you can enjoy them without overindulging.

- Avoid the buffet table. Find someone to visit with who is sitting far away from the food. Focus on conversation, not eating.

- Keep a glass of water or diet soda in your hands. This will keep one fewer hand out of the high-calorie goodies.

- Bring a healthy appetizer like raw veggies or fruit to ensure that you will have something to snack on that supports your healthy habits.

The Party's Over

- If you end up with leftovers that are tempting, send them home with your guests or share them with an elderly friend or family member.

- Freeze some of the leftovers in single servings to take for lunches or to have for dinners on the run.

- In preparation for the new year, purge your pantry of any junk foods or tempting foods. Out with the old, in with the new!

A New Beginning

- Greet the new year with a healthy attitude. Write one goal for the year in each of these areas: spiritual, emotional, mental and physical.

- Start the new year off by planning your first week of menus along with your shopping list.

- Renew your subscriptions to any health newsletters or magazines for the coming year, or sign up to receive free health and fitness email newsletters or other publications.

NO-WORRY THANKSGIVING!
by Scott Wilson

- Before the big day, experiment with recipes in order to familiarize yourself with their preparation. Get everything out on the counter and ready to go.

- As much as possible, try to prepare things ahead of time. For example, homemade cranberry sauce tastes better after curing it in the refrigerator for a few days; pre-measure seasonings and store them in labeled bags or containers; clean, cut and store vegetables in plastic bags in the refrigerator.

- Let your family set the table. Children will gobble up the chance to make place cards, fold napkins and dress up the holiday table. This will also keep them out of the kitchen while you attend to the food.

- Serve buffet-style. With pretty serving bowls and silver utensils, guests can help themselves to seconds whenever they want, while you remember your portion sizes.

- Let the turkey rest before slicing. To avoid a last-minute crunch and assure tender turkey, let the bird rest out of the oven, covered, for about 30 minutes before slicing.

- Use your microwave oven. Take advantage of this appliance so that you can quickly reheat food before serving when all the burners on the stovetop are occupied.

- Thermometers are essential for food safety. When choosing a meat thermometer, look for an easy-to-read dial with a stainless-steel face and shatterproof lens. Check the thermometer for accuracy by submerging at least two inches of the stem in boiling water. It should read 212° F (or the boiling temperature of water at your altitude). An alternative to the typical meat thermometer is an instant-read thermometer (also known as a rapid-response thermometer), which is designed to measure a wide range of temperatures, typically from 0° F to 220° F. It does not stay in food during cooking. When it's inserted in the food, the temperature registers in about 15 seconds.

- Finally, remember that this is Thanksgiving! Take time to thank God for what He has done in your life this past year and for what He is going to do for you in the coming year.

CHRISTMAS MISSION: POSSIBLE

*And let us consider how we may spur one
another on toward love and good deeds.*
HEBREWS 10:24

*Jesus looked at them and said, "With man this is impossible,
but with God all things are possible."*
MATTHEW 19:26

Dear Family,

I have thought about our Christmas this year
and wondered what would give it more fullness.
It seems that when we help someone else, we
gain pleasure and satisfaction and become better
people. Our happiness is not always just a result
of getting something. We all have so very many
good things. Could we share our gifts this year
with others?

This year, I am challenging you—should you choose
to accept this mission—to take the enclosed
Christmas check and decide how best to use it.
After considering the possibilities, you may:

- Buy something for yourself.

- Use a portion of it to buy yourself what you
  want and the other portion to share with another person who has less or who needs help.

- Work together with other family members to
  complete a project.

When we get together for Christmas, please bring all of your gifts to open that day. Wrap the gift for yourself. Wrap the gift that you are sharing with someone else. If you have already given them the gift, put something in the box that tells the story of your gift to share with the rest of us.

I love you all and look forward to a special time together at Christmas this year.

Blessings.

P.S. Some ideas:

1. Volunteer to serve a holiday meal to needy families.

2. Give a gift to someone in another country through Heifer International (www.heifer.org) or Samaritan's Purse (www.samaritanspurse.org).

3. Send cards to military service personnel. Access www.anysoldier.com for further information.

4. THE American Legion takes gift donations for American soldiers who get few letters and gifts and are serving in other countries.

5. Give donations to a food pantry.

6. Find a project in your church or community.

7. Donate time and/or gifts to a nonprofit group.

HEALTHY HOLIDAY COOKING HINTS

- Purchase a turkey without added fat; that is, those that have butter or oil injected under the skin.

- If you use broth from the turkey, remove the fat. This can be done by allowing the broth to cool in the refrigerator or by skimming the broth with ice cubes.

- Quick and easy pies can be made from instant or cook-and-serve sugar-free pudding. Any flavor fruit pie can be made by using fresh fruit such as apples or peaches. Slice fruit, place in a saucepan, add a cup of apple juice or other fruit juice and one cup of water; cook until softened. Sweeten to taste with artificial sweetener. Add spices, if desired, and thicken with cornstarch. You now have a sugar-free, fat-free filling.

- Applesauce is a great substitute for fat and sugar in recipes. You can exchange a half cup of applesauce for a half cup of oil or for a half cup of sugar. (*Note:* Substantial amounts of substitutes for the sugar and oil do not exchange well. That is why it is best to only replace part of the sugar or oil.)

- The holiday season is a good time to experiment with dips. Use plain yogurt instead of sour cream. Even though the fat-free sour cream is devoid of fat grams, it is also devoid of nutrients. Keep in mind that our goal is to eat foods with as many nutrients as possible.

- Add yogurt mixed with fruit to Jell-O for a creamy dessert.

BRING JOY TO THE SEASON

- Send Christmas notes to at least six people who blessed you this past year. For example: Thank your First Place 4 Health leader or a member who has encouraged you. Be specific about how they helped you.

- Call someone who may be having a sad holiday and let them know you are thinking of them, such as a friend who had a death in the family during the year or someone who is ill.

- Invite someone to be a part of your holiday celebration who would have little family activity otherwise. For example: Take that person to a church party or to look at Christmas lights.

- Make a spiritual event part of your Christmas tradition. For example: Read the Christmas story in Matthew 1:18-25, Luke 2:1-20 and Matthew 2:1-12, or attend a candlelight service or church pageant.

- Tell stories of family Christmases past. Find visual reminders such as old decorations, cards, photos or gifts of past Christmases that you have experienced. Share stories that older relatives have told about their Christmases. Heirloom stories tie families to their heritage and encourage them to make memories for the future.

- Mail New Year's greetings to as many friends and family as possible. The time after Christmas is often a period when you can have more time to be reflective, and New Year's notes are less likely to be lost in all the Christmas mail.

- *Slow down*, take a deep breath and plan a successful and meaningful holiday. *Drop* the unimportant, even if others want to pressure you. *Add* the important, even if no one but you finds meaning in it. *Enjoy* people more than things and the gift of the Son of God more than anything else! When He is in first place, all the season's events hold the potential for joy.

AVOID EMOTIONAL TRAPS

- Comparison. Festive outings can often be occasions for being placed in uncomfortable situations that give rise to feelings of inferiority, embarrassment or shame. This may occur at company dinners, family gatherings or church parties where poise and physical appearance seem to be more important than ever. These situations may stir up past feelings of not measuring up that can date back to a childhood party or an embarrassing blunder in a Christmas play. When you begin to feel inferior or ashamed, it's time to remind yourself what God's Word says about you! Memorize Scripture verses that will arm you with truthful encouragement when you are tempted to compare.

- Expectations. For many people, the holidays are not emotional lifts; they are emotional downers. All the celebration makes tough times seem tougher and sad times seem sadder, often because people expect to be filled with joy. Sometimes we have idealized expectations for holiday events that are not based in reality, and when those expectations are not met, we become depressed. Learn to be realistic about your expectations, and don't punish yourself if you are having a difficult time. Draw close to God and ask Him to soothe your troubled spirit.

- Difficult Settings. Perhaps unlike any other time of the year, the time between Thanksgiving and New Year's Day draws more families together than at any other time. If family gatherings are affirming, they can be an emotionally positive time. But for millions of people, the holidays are filled with past pain, guilt, unresolved anger, destructive secrets and old unhealthy patterns. Painful family situations include a divorced couple splitting Christmas with the children, or an adult visiting an overly controlling mother, an alcoholic father or an out-of-control sibling. In order to minimize the negative influence of holiday distractions to healthy living, it is important to increase the positive factors.

- Evaluate. Looking back on the past few holiday seasons, consider what caused pain and what caused joy. Add more of the joy factors (for example, sponsoring a needy family or attending a Christmas Eve service). Attempt to discover patterns of pain, and make plans to minimize their impact before they occur (for example, keeping your visit short or putting off a visit until a less stressful time).

- Plan and Get Support. Don't just let the holidays sweep you along. Plan now what you will or won't do. Seek the support of at least two people to be your reality check and prayer-support partners. They can give their impression of what is a reasonable or healthy reaction to low self-esteem issues or painful family situations.

Light & Healthy Holidays
leader discussion guide

The First Place 4 Health holiday session is six weeks long with one group meeting per week, and is recommended for any member who has completed at least one regular First Place 4 Health session. This shorter session is specially designed for First Place 4 Health members who desire to maintain their healthy habits during the holidays.

Each group meeting should last approximately one hour, with 15-minute segments set aside for (1) weigh-in and memory verse recitation, (2) Wellness Spotlight, (3) devotion/journal discussion, and (4) prayer requests and prayer. Before the first meeting, your group members should memorize the Week One memory verse as they read the daily devotions, complete the journaling assignments, and complete the prayer partner form to turn in during class. They should also fill out their Live It Tracker each day and turn it in at the group meeting. (See the *First Place 4 Health Leader's Guide* for tips on how to evaluate your members' Live It Trackers.)

Following is a suggested outline for each of the six group meetings.

WEEK ONE: GIVING THANKS
Weigh-in and Memory Verse (15 minutes)
Weigh and measure members and listen as they recite the week's Scripture memory verse.

Wellness Spotlight (15 minutes)

Staying motivated during the holidays can be especially difficult, but staying motivated can be difficult at any time of the year if one loses sight of how he or she can benefit from his or her weight-loss efforts. Ask members to share their answers to the following:

1. Have you ever gained weight during the holidays?
2. What tempts you to overeat?
3. What's the payoff when you overeat? What do you get out of overeating?
4. What might you gain by staying focused during the holidays?

Guide your members to make realistic goals for the holiday session. Have them discuss in small groups or with the whole group some strategies that may keep them focused on their holiday goals.

List these strategies on a whiteboard, chalkboard or poster board. If they have not yet done so, have them complete the goal-making exercise in the introduction of this book.

Devotion/Journal Discussion (15 minutes)

Invite volunteers to share about losses they have experienced, and then list any blessings that have come from the loss.

Ask members to share Scripture verses that have brought comfort or healing to their life.

Prayer Requests/Prayer (15 minutes)

Have members write a praise or something for which they are thankful on small index cards. Send a basket around and fill it with the blessings.

For the prayer time, read the praises, and then ask each member to pray by speaking a one-word praise (e.g., children, health, Jesus).

Before the group leaves, pass around the basket for prayer partner forms. Have each member draw a form from the basket on his or her way out.

WEEK TWO: GOODNESS AND LOVE
Memory Verse (15 minutes)
Listen as the members in your group recite the current week's Scripture memory verse.

Wellness Spotlight (15 minutes)
Each of your group members will certainly want to survive the holidays with his or her healthy habits still in place. So, for this session, you will begin to plan activities with your group that will take them through the holidays and enable them to become healthier physically, emotionally, mentally and spiritually in the coming year.

Before the meeting, call members and ask them to bring a day-planner or PDA to the meeting. Ask members to split into pairs and review "Holiday Survival Tips" in Holiday Helps, selecting one activity for each week from the list. Have them write that activity on a specific date of their calendar, noting whether it is aimed at their physical, spiritual, emotional or mental health.

Invite partners to pray for each other during the meeting about the activities they have chosen and keep each other accountable in the coming weeks.

Having your members anticipate challenges or obstacles that they will face on Thanksgiving will allow them time to develop strategies to overcome these challenges. Instruct members to write out what they plan to eat on Thanksgiving Day. Refer them to the 1,400-calorie Thanksgiving Day menu and to the recipes that follow, as well as to "No-Worry Thanksgiving" in the Holiday Helps.

Ask members to share the strategies they plan to use to overcome some of the challenges that this holiday will bring. Refer them to "Holiday Survival Tips" in Holiday Helps for ideas.

Devotion/Journal Discussion (15 minutes)

Ask members to list character traits of God. Then have volunteers explain how they have come to know more fully a specific character trait of God.

Write Psalm 139:14 on a whiteboard, chalkboard or poster board and display it in the room. Ask volunteers who have memorized the verse to quote it for the group. Then have each member tell one wonderful way God has created him or her (for example, strong legs, excellent vision, a good singing voice).

Prayer Requests/Prayer (15 minutes)

Pray aloud in unison using Psalm 139:14 and then have volunteers pray and thank God for His wonderful works.

Before the group leaves, pass around the basket for prayer partner forms. Have each member draw a form from the basket on his or her way out.

WEEK THREE: GREAT JOY

Memory Verse (15 minutes)

Listen as the members in your group recite the current week's Scripture memory verse.

Wellness Spotlight (15 minutes)

Ask members to consider how focusing on giving to others can help them maintain their fitness goals. Refer them to "Christmas Mission: Possible" in Holiday Helps and lead a discussion about the pros and cons of this mission idea. Would doing it help to put the focus on Christ and others instead of self? Would members' families have problems adjusting to the idea? Why or why not?

Devotion/Journal Discussion (15 minutes)

Before the meeting, call a member and ask him or her to prepare to give a brief (5 to 6 minutes) testimony of his or her salvation. Begin the devotion/journal discussion by inviting this member to share.

Ask members, "What is your focus during this holiday?" Invite volunteers to share how they (as an individual or as a family) keep their focus on the birth of Christ rather than on buying gifts.

Discuss all of the roles that they take on, such as mom, dad, sister, wife, volunteer, Sunday School teacher, choir member, and so on during this busy season.

As a group, read Isaiah 9:6 aloud, and then list the names of Jesus that are stated in this verse. Ask members which name they need to call on to meet the needs of a specific responsibility that they must fulfill.

Prayer Requests/Prayer (15 minutes)

Invite members to pray aloud short prayers that use the names of Jesus from Isaiah 9:6.

Before the group leaves, pass around the basket for prayer partner forms. Have each member draw a form from the basket on his or her way out.

Note: For next week's meeting, invite volunteers to bring in a holiday party food, such as a dip, finger food or treat, using one of the holiday recipes or one of their own light recipes. If they bring a recipe of their own, ask them to provide copies of the recipe for the other members.

Optional: Have a recipe exchange. Invite members to bring copies of at least one light-eating recipe to share with others.

WEEK FOUR: COME TO WORSHIP
Memory Verse (15 minutes)
Listen as the members in your group recite the current week's Scripture memory verse.

Wellness Spotlight (15 minutes)
In this session, you will experiment with healthy holiday recipes. Read through "Healthy Holiday Cooking Hints" in Holiday Helps, and ask members to share ideas for lightening up their favorite holiday recipes.

Discuss the 1,400-calorie Christmas menu and recipes and how they plan on utilizing this tool as they plan their Christmas menu.

Optional: Allow time for members to exchange their light holiday recipes while tasting the foods that were brought to class.

Devotion/Journal Discussion (15 minutes)
Ask members to share with the group how God has shown His love to them this week.

Brainstorm ways that they can show God's love to their neighbors or to the hard-to-love people in their lives.

Prayer Requests/Prayer (15 minutes)
Read Ephesians 3:16-19. Invite members to pray this Scripture for one another before closing in prayer.

Before the group leaves, pass around the basket for prayer partner forms. Have each member draw a form from the basket on his or her way out.

WEEK FIVE: BE MADE NEW
Memory Verse (15 minutes)

Listen as the members in your group recite the current week's Scripture memory verse.

Wellness Spotlight (15 minutes)

In this session, the group will focus on spreading joy to others. Before the meeting, gather blank cards and other supplies (construction paper, stickers, rubber stamps and stamp pads, felt-tip pens, glue and so forth) to make greeting cards.

If you have a member who is good with crafts, you can enlist his or her help in showing members how to make a specific type of card—but keep it simple!

Have each member select one person they want to encourage. Have each member send that person a special New Year's card. Invite volunteers to share about their card's recipient and why they chose that person.

Ask members to plan their New Year's Day menu by using the 1,400-calorie New Year's Day menu and recipes.

Devotion/Journal Discussion (15 minutes)

Give each member a blank piece of paper and ask them to list anything in their past that they would consider a failure. Have them each silently ask God to forgive them for their part in the failure, and then ask Him to make a way for them to correct the failure and leave the incident in the past.

After a few minutes of private prayer, have members tear up their paper and throw it in the trash (or have a paper shredder handy for this task). This is a way of putting their failures in the past and forgetting them.

Optional: If you have a safe way to do this (i.e., a fireplace or outdoor barbeque or fire ring), invite members to burn the paper to signify that their failures are forgiven and forgotten by God.

Invite members to share their dreams for the new year by sharing what new thing they would like to accomplish.

Prayer Requests/Prayer (15 minutes)

Invite members to share the areas of commitment or situations in which they need God's power to accomplish a miracle. Pray Isaiah 48:14, that God would make a way through their specific situations.

Before the group leaves, pass around the basket for prayer partner forms. Have each member draw a form from the basket on his or her way out.

WEEK SIX: A NEW HEART

Weigh-in and Memory Verse (15 minutes)

Weigh and measure members and listen as they recite the week's Scripture memory verse.

Wellness Spotlight (15 minutes)

The holidays can be full of joy, but they can also bring many stresses. It is important your group members learn to manage these negative influences in their lives in order to maintain a healthy and balanced life. Reflecting on this holiday season, ask your group what they can do differently next year to avoid emotional traps.

Have members form pairs and share about holiday stressors. If they feel comfortable, ask them to reflect on any particular days or people that caused them to be especially emotional during the holiday season.

As they review "Avoid Emotional Traps" in the Holiday Helps, ask them to plan for next year by evaluating what they could have done differently. Have partners pray for one another.

Devotion/Journal Discussion

Invite members to share about some old things that they need to get rid of this year (attitudes, habits, possessions and so forth).

Explain that 2 Corinthians 5:17 suggests that we must "put on" the new self. Invite members to share about how they plan to put on a new self physically, spiritually, emotionally and mentally.

Have members brainstorm ways that they can support one another to remain faithful to their First Place 4 Health commitment.

Challenge members to bring friends to the next orientation meeting to get the new year off to a great start!

Prayer Requests/Prayer (15 minutes)

Invite members to divide into pairs for a time of prayer. Have each partner pray for the other, asking God to bless them in the coming year and to give them strength to put Him first in their lives.

Before the group leaves, pass around the basket for prayer partner forms. Have each member draw a form from the basket on his or her way out.

First Place 4 Health
holiday menus & recipes

Each menu plan is based on approximately 1,400 calories. The nutritional information for these meals was calculated using the MasterCook software. It uses a database of over 6,000 food items prepared using United States Department of Agriculture (USDA) publications and information from food manufacturers. As with any nutritional program, MasterCook calculates the nutritional values of the recipes based on ingredients. Nutrition may vary due to how the food is prepared, where the food comes from, soil content, season, ripeners, and processing and methods of preparation. For these reasons, please use the recipes and menu plans as approximate guides. As always, consult your physician and/or registered dietitian before starting a diet program.

For those who need more calories, add the following to the 1,400-calorie plan:

- 1,800 calories: 2 ounce equivalent of meat, 3 ounce equivalent of bread, 1/2 cup vegetable serving, 1 tsp. fat

- 2,000 calories: 2 ounce equivalent of meat, 4 ounce equivalent of bread, 1/2 cup vegetable serving, 3 tsp. fat

- 2,200 calories: 2 ounce equivalent of meat, 5 ounce equivalent of bread, 1/2 cup vegetable serving, 1/2 cup fruit serving, 5 tsp. fat

- 2,400 calories: 2 ounce equivalent of meat, 6 ounce equivalent of bread, 1 cup vegetable serving, 1/2 cup fruit serving, 6 tsp. fat

Thanksgiving Day Menus and Recipes

Note: Recipes for items *italicized in bold* are included below.

MENUS

Breakfast

1 cup nonfat milk   ¹/₂ cup bran flake cereal

1¹/₄ cups strawberries
    (or other fruit)

Nutritional Information: 219 calories; 2g fat (7% calories from fat); 12g protein; 44g carbohydrate; 8g dietary fiber; 4mg cholesterol; 301mg sodium.

Thanksgiving Meal

1 (4 oz.) serving *Roast Turkey*   1 cup *Spicy Fresh Green Beans*
    with Herbs   ¹/₂ cup *Broccoli Rice Casserole*

1 cup *Cornbread Dressing*   ¹/₂ cup *Cranberry Gelatin Salad*

2 tbsp. *Creamy Gravy*   ¹/₈ slice *Pumpkin Soufflé*

Nutritional Information: 719 calories; 23g fat (30% calories from fat); 6g saturated fat; 9g monounsaturated fat; 5g polyunsaturated fat; 50g protein; 77g carbohydrate; 9g dietary fiber; 169mg cholesterol; 1,670mg sodium.

Dinner

(May be used for lunch or dinner.)

1 *Turkey Philly*   Fresh fruit with

1 cup carrot and celery sticks with   1 cup fat-free yogurt
    1 tbsp. low-fat Ranch dressing

Nutritional Information: 474 calories; 12g fat (23% calories from fat); 6g saturated fat; 39g protein; 55g carbohydrate; 6g dietary fiber; 74mg cholesterol; 1,246mg sodium.

RECIPES
Roast Turkey with Herbs

Note: If you are using a frozen turkey, allow 3 to 4 days for the turkey to thaw in the refrigerator; do not thaw at room temperature.

$^1/_4$ cup minced onion

$^1/_2$ tsp. dried leaf thyme

$^1/_2$ tsp. dried rubbed sage

3 tbsp. grated lemon rind

$^1/_2$ cup chicken broth

2 cups chicken or turkey broth

10 to 12 lbs. turkey (completely thawed if frozen)

Nonstick cooking spray

Preheat oven to 400° F. Combine onion, thyme, sage, lemon rind and chicken broth. Remove giblets from turkey cavity and discard; rinse turkey and pat dry. Lift skin away from turkey breast and spread mixture between skin and turkey. Use any remaining herb mixture inside turkey cavity. Place turkey on rack that has been sprayed with nonstick cooking spray; put rack in roasting pan and pour broth around turkey. Roast turkey at 400° F for 30 minutes. Reduce oven temperature to 350° F; continue roasting until meat thermometer inserted into thickest part of thigh registers 175° F, about 2 hours. (Baste every 30 minutes, if desired.) Transfer turkey to platter; tent with foil and let stand 30 minutes before slicing to let juices set. Serving size: 4 ounces. Serves 15 to 20.

Nutritional Information: 287 calories; 14g fat (46% calories from fat); 4g saturated fat; 5g monounsaturated fat; 3g polyunsaturated fat; 37g protein; 1g carbohydrate; trace dietary fiber; 140mg cholesterol; 206mg sodium.

Cornbread Dressing

1 (8-oz.) pkg. herb-seasoned
   cornbread stuffing mix
2 (6-oz.) pkg. cornbread mix
2 whole eggs
1$^1/_3$ cups skim milk
1$^1/_2$ cups onion, chopped

1$^1/_2$ cups celery, chopped
10 chicken bouillon cubes
10 cups water
1 tbsp. poultry seasoning
4 egg whites

Make cornbread according to package directions, using the 2 whole eggs and skim milk. Boil celery, onion and bouillon cubes in water over low heat for 3 to 5 minutes. Crumble cooked cornbread and combine with stuffing mix. Pour boiled mixture over bread mixture. After mixture has cooled, stir in beaten egg whites. Bake in two pans at 375° F for 1$^1/_2$ hours. Serves 16.

Nutritional Information: 178 calories; 4g fat (21% calories from fat); 1g saturated fat; 2g monounsaturated fat; 1g polyunsaturated fat; 6g protein; 29g carbohydrate; 3g dietary fiber; 28mg cholesterol; 952mg sodium.

Creamy Gravy

4 chicken bouillon cubes
3 cups water

2 tbsp. flour
Salt and pepper to taste

Add bouillon to water boiling in large saucepan. In a pint jar with lid, combine $^3/_4$ cup of bouillon water with flour; shake well. Slowly pour into remaining water, stirring constantly to prevent lumps. Simmer over low heat, stirring frequently until gravy consistency is reached. Add flour or water if needed to reach desired consistency. Add salt and pepper to taste. Serves 16.

Nutritional Information: 6 calories; trace fat (22% calories from fat); trace protein; 1g carbohydrate; trace dietary fiber; trace cholesterol; 187mg sodium.

Spicy Fresh Green Beans

2 lbs. fresh green beans, cleaned
  and snapped at both ends
1 large onion, sliced
1 tbsp. minced garlic
1 tbsp. cracked black pepper

1 tbsp. Tony Chachere's seasoning
Salt to taste
6 chicken bouillon cubes
6 to 8 fresh new potatoes,
  if desired

Place first six ingredients in large stock pan. Add water 4 inches above beans. Add 6 squares chicken bouillon to water. Cook over medium heat (low boil) until beans are tender, 1 to 2 hours. Add more water as needed. Add 6 to 8 small fresh new potatoes after 1 hour of cooking, if desired. Prick potatoes with a fork to check if done. Serves 8.

Nutritional Information (without potatoes): 39 calories; trace fat (3% calories from fat); 2g protein; 9g carbohydrate; 4g dietary fiber; 0mg cholesterol; 7mg sodium.

Broccoli Rice Casserole

$1^1/_2$ cups uncooked rice
$^1/_2$ cup chopped onion
$^1/_2$ cup chopped celery
$^1/_2$ cup light margarine

1 can Healthy Request Cream
  of Mushroom Soup
1 (8-oz.) jar Cheez Whiz Light
1 (10-oz.) bag broccoli florets

Cook rice as directed for half the time indicated. While rice is cooking, sauté onion and celery in margarine until soft, about 5 minutes. Add Cheez Whiz and stir until melted. Add Cream of Mushroom soup and stir until thoroughly mixed. Fold in broccoli florets. Pour into 13 x 9 casserole pan. Bake in 350° F oven until bubbly and lightly browned on top, about 30 to 45 minutes. Serves 12.

Nutritional Information: 128 calories; 4g fat (28% calories from fat); 1g saturated fat; 2g monounsaturated fat; 1g polyunsaturated fat; 3g protein; 21g carbohydrate; 1g dietary fiber; trace cholesterol; 106mg sodium.

Cranberry Gelatin Salad

2 (3-oz.) pkg. sugar-free
cranberry gelatin
1³/₄ cups boiling water
³/₄ cup cold water
³/₄ cup red delicious
apple, diced

³/₄ cup golden delicious
apple, diced
¹/₂ cup green seedless grapes,
halved
¹/₄ cup chopped pecans (optional)
Cooking spray

Put dry gelatin in a medium bowl. Pour in boiling water; stir for 2 minutes. Stir in cold water. Add diced apples and grapes. Mix well. Pour into 13 x 9 pan sprayed with cooking spray. Refrigerate until set. Garnish with chopped pecans if desired. Serves 8.

Nutritional Information (without pecans): 14 calories; trace fat (3% calories from fat); trace protein; 4g carbohydrate; 1g dietary fiber; 0mg cholesterol; 3mg sodium.

Creamy Pumpkin Soufflé

1 (1.5-oz.) box sugar-free vanilla-
flavored nonfat instant pudding
1 cup nonfat milk
1 (16-oz.) can pumpkin

¹/₂ tsp. nutmeg
¹/₂ tsp. ginger
¹/₂ tsp. cinnamon
1 cup Cool Whip Lite

Combine pudding mix and milk in medium bowl; stir well. Add pumpkin, nutmeg, ginger and cinnamon; stir. Gently fold in whipped topping. Pour into pudding cups. Chill for one hour or until set. Serves 8.

Nutritional Information: 65 calories; 1g fat (16% calories from fat); 2g protein; 12g carbohydrate; trace dietary fiber; 1mg cholesterol; 124mg sodium.

Turkey Philly

1 cup thinly sliced onion
1 cup thinly sliced green
bell pepper

¹/₄ tsp. black pepper
³/₄ lb. thinly sliced deli
turkey breast

2 tsp. butter

4 (2-oz.) sandwich rolls

4 (1-oz.) slices low-sodium
mozzarella or provolone cheese

Preheat oven to 375° F. Melt butter in a large nonstick skillet over medium-high heat. Add onion and bell pepper; sauté 5 minutes or until tender. Stir in black pepper. Divide onion mixture and turkey evenly among bottom halves of rolls; top each serving with 1 cheese slice. Cover with top halves of rolls. Place sandwiches on a baking sheet. Bake at 375° F for 5 minutes or until cheese melts. Serves 4.

Nutritional Information: 292 calories; 11g fat (33% calories from fat); 6g saturated fat; 25g protein; 25g carbohydrate; 2g dietary fiber; 70mg cholesterol; 1,027mg sodium.

ADDITIONAL THANKSGIVING RECIPES

Turkey Bolognese

1/4 cup extra-virgin olive oil

1 onion, chopped

4 garlic cloves, minced

1 carrot, peeled and finely chopped

1 celery stalk, finely chopped

1 lb. shredded cooked turkey
(preferably dark meat)

3 cups marinara sauce

1/4 cup chopped fresh basil leaves

Salt and freshly ground
black pepper

1 pound spaghetti

Freshly grated Parmesan cheese

Heat oil in a large heavy frying pan over medium heat. Add onion and garlic and sauté until translucent, about 5 minutes. Add carrot and celery and sauté until vegetables are tender, about 5 minutes. Add turkey and sauté 1 minute. Add marinara sauce. Decrease heat to medium-low and simmer for 15 minutes to allow flavors to blend, stirring often. Stir in basil. Season sauce to taste with salt and pepper. (Sauce can be made 1 week ahead. Cool completely after preparation, then transfer to a container and freeze for future use. Bring sauce to a simmer before using.)

Meanwhile, cook spaghetti in a large pot of boiling salted water, stirring often, about 8 minutes or until just tender but still firm to bite. Drain, reserving 1 cup of cooking liquid. Add pasta to sauce and toss to coat, adding enough reserved cooking liquid to moisten as needed. Serve with Parmesan cheese. Serves 4.

Nutritional Information: 432 calories; 12g fat (26% calories from fat); 2g saturated fat; 6g monounsaturated fat; 2g polyunsaturated fat; 26g protein; 53g carbohydrate; 4g dietary fiber; 43mg cholesterol; 438mg sodium.

Sweet Potato Casserole

3 lbs. sweet potatoes

$1/3$ cup packed brown sugar

2 tbsp. butter

2 tbsp. orange juice concentrate

$1^1/2$ tsp. ground cinnamon

$1/2$ tsp. salt

$1/2$ tsp. ground nutmeg

2 large eggs

$1/4$ cup chopped pecans

Preheat oven to 350° F. Pierce potatoes several times with a fork; arrange in a circle on paper towels in microwave oven. Microwave on High for 16 minutes or until tender, rearranging potatoes after 8 minutes. Let stand 5 minutes. Cut each potato in half lengthwise; scoop out pulp into a large bowl. Discard skins.

Add sugar, butter, orange juice concentrate, cinnamon and nutmeg, and beat with a mixer at low speed until combined. Add eggs and beat until smooth. Spoon mixture into a $1^1/2$ quart baking dish and sprinkle with pecans. Bake at 350° F for 45 minutes or until thoroughly heated. Serves 8.

Nutritional Information: 241 calories; 7g fat (25% calories from fat); 2g saturated fat; 3g monounsaturated fat; 1g polyunsaturated fat; 4g protein; 42g carbohydrate; 4g dietary fiber; 61mg cholesterol; 200mg sodium.

Cranberry Apple Relish

1¹/₂ cups chopped, peeled Granny
  Smith apples (about ¹/₂ lb.)
1 cup packed brown sugar
¹/₂ cup white grape juice

1 tsp. ground ginger
1 tsp. ground cinnamon
1 (12-oz.) package fresh
  cranberries

Combine all ingredients in a medium saucepan. Bring to a boil; reduce heat and simmer until thick (about 15 minutes), stirring occasionally. Cool completely or chill before serving. Serves 16.

Nutritional Information: 61 calories; trace fat; trace protein; 16g carbohydrate; trace dietary fiber; 0mg cholesterol; 6mg sodium.

Christmas Day Menus and Recipes

Note: Recipes for items *italicized in bold* are included below.

MENUS

Breakfast

1 *Tropical Muffin*   1 cup mixed fruit
1 cup nonfat milk

Nutritional Information: 278 calories; 5g fat (34% calories from fat); 2g saturated fat; 1g monounsaturated fat; 1g polyunsaturated fat; 12g protein; 48g carbohydrate; 4g dietary fiber; 22mg cholesterol; 391mg sodium.

Christmas Meal

4 oz. *Golden Fruited Ham*   2 cups mixed greens salad
$1/4$ cup *Cinnamon Apples*   with 1 tbsp. light dressing
1 cup green beans $1/8$ *Lemon Icebox Dessert*

Nutritional Information: 575 calories; 9g fat (15% calories from fat); 2g saturated fat; 4g monounsaturated fat; 1g polyunsaturated fat; 38g protein; 84g carbohydrate; 10g dietary fiber; 83mg cholesterol; 2,721mg sodium.

Dinner

(May be used for lunch or dinner.)

1 serving *Hearty Vegetable Soup*   1 tbsp. salad dressing
2 cups large green salad topped   3 crackers
   with 1 oz. turkey, cubed   1 serving *Fruit Breeze*

Nutritional Information: 401 calories; 10g fat (23% calories from fat); 2g saturated fat; 19g protein; 58g carbohydrate; 8g dietary fiber; 13mg cholesterol; 1,127mg sodium.

RECIPES

Tropical Muffins

1¹/₄ cups flour

³/₄ cup sugar substitute

2 tsp. baking powder

¹/₄ tsp. baking soda

¹/₂ tsp. salt

¹/₄ cup unsweetened
   coconut flakes

3 ripe bananas, mashed

¹/₃ cup reduced-fat
   margarine, melted

1 egg, beaten

1 tsp. grated orange rind

¹/₃ cup unsweetened orange juice

Nonstick cooking spray

Preheat oven to 375° F. Sift together flour, sugar substitute, baking powder, baking soda and salt in large bowl. Stir in coconut and form a well in center of mixture, set aside. In separate bowl, combine bananas, margarine, egg, orange rind and orange juice. Mix well and pour into dry ingredients well, stirring until dry ingredients are just moistened. Spoon batter into muffin pan coated with cooking spray, filling cups ²/₃ full. Bake 25 to 30 minutes or until lightly browned. Serves 12.

Nutritional Information: 127 calories; 4g fat (29% calories from fat); 2g saturated fat; 1g monounsaturated fat; 1g polyunsaturated fat; 3g protein; 20g carbohydrate; 1g dietary fiber; 18mg cholesterol; 265mg sodium.

Golden Fruited Ham

2 lbs. extra-lean reduced-sodium
   ham, sliced and trimmed of fat

1 (12-oz.) jar all-fruit apricot
   spread preserves

1 tbsp. Dijon mustard

¹/₂ tsp. ground ginger

¹/₈ tsp. ground cloves

¹/₂ cup raisins

$1/4$ cup firmly packed light
  brown sugar
2 tbsp. flour
1 tbsp. white wine vinegar

1 (15-oz.) can apricot halves,
  drained and coarsely chopped
2 tbsp. cornstarch
2 tbsp. water

Trim fat from ham; place in 4-quart electric slow-cooker. In large bowl, combine preserves, brown sugar, flour, vinegar, mustard, ginger and cloves; stir well. Add apricots and raisins; stir well and pour over ham. Cover cooker with lid; cook on High for 2 hours or until ham is thoroughly heated. Remove meat from cooker; set aside and keep warm. Pour cooking liquid into small saucepan; set aside. Combine cornstarch and water in small bowl; stir until smooth. Add to cooking liquid; bring to a boil and cook 1 minute or until thick, stirring constantly. Serve about $1/4$ cup of sauce with each 4-oz. ham serving. Serves 6.

Nutritional Information: 311 calories; 8g fat (23% calories from fat); 2g saturated fat; 4g monounsaturated fat; 1g polyunsaturated fat; 30g protein; 29g carbohydrate; 1g dietary fiber; 71mg cholesterol; 2,200mg sodium.

Cinnamon Apples

6 cups chopped, peeled Granny
  Smith apples (about 2 lbs.)
$1/2$ cup packed brown sugar
$1/4$ cup apple juice

1 tsp. ground cinnamon
$1/8$ tsp. ground nutmeg
$1/8$ tsp. salt

Combine all ingredients in a large heavy saucepan. Cover and cook over medium-low heat for 45 minutes or until apples are tender, stirring occasionally. Let stand 5 minutes. Serves 8.

Nutritional Information: 121 calories; trace protein; 0mg cholesterol; 19mg calcium; 2g dietary fiber; trace iron; 31g carbohydrate; 42mg sodium.

Lemon Icebox Dessert

1 (1.5-oz.) box sugar-free vanilla-
flavored nonfat instant pudding

$1/2$ (.8 g.) container Crystal Light
sugar-free lemonade drink mix

6 low-fat graham crackers

2 cups nonfat milk

3 cups fat-free whipped topping

Line bottom of 11 x 7 baking dish with graham crackers; set aside. In a large bowl, use electric mixer on low speed to blend together pudding mix, lemonade mix and milk. Use spatula or wooden spoon to fold in $2^1/_4$ cups of whipped topping. Pour mixture over graham crackers, top with remaining whipped topping. Refrigerate until ready to serve, at least one hour. Serves 8.

Nutritional Information: 80 calories; 1g fat (12% calories from fat); 3g protein; 11g carbohydrate; trace dietary fiber; 1mg cholesterol; 95mg sodium.

Hearty Vegetable Soup

2 cups frozen mixed vegetables

2 cans beef broth

1 can vegetable broth

1 can chicken broth

1 (15-oz.) can chopped tomatoes

4 medium potatoes, cut into pieces

$1^1/_2$ cups sliced carrots

$1/_4$ head cabbage, sliced

1 medium onion, chopped

Basil and bay leaf to taste,
dried or fresh

Mix all ingredients together in a large pot. Simmer until vegetables are tender. Serving size: 1 cup. Serves 10.

Nutritional Information: 91 calories; 1g fat (7% calories from fat); 5g protein; 17g carbohydrate; 2g dietary fiber; trace cholesterol; 509mg sodium.

Berry Breeze

1 (8-oz.) container Cool
Whip Lite

2 (6-oz.) containers light
berry-flavored yogurt

2 cups fresh berries (strawberries,   1 reduced-fat graham cracker
  blueberries, raspberries)   crust

Mix all together and pour into crust. Refrigerate for at least 30 minutes, slice and serve. Serves 8.

Nutritional Information: 211 calories; 7g fat (33% calories from fat); 2g saturated fat; 4g protein; 29g carbohydrate; 2g dietary fiber; 1mg cholesterol; 67mg sodium.

To make individual servings of Berry Breeze, place 1 tbsp. graham cracker crumbs in each of 8 serving dishes and top with 1/2 cup berries. Mix yogurt and Cool Whip together, and spoon over berries. Refrigerate for at least 30 minutes and serve garnished with a berry.

Nutritional Information: 144 calories; 4g fat (29% calories from fat); 3g protein; 21g carbohydrate; 2g dietary fiber; 1mg cholesterol; 87mg sodium.

ADDITIONAL CHRISTMAS RECIPES
Sugar-Free Spiced Tea Mix
Note: Great idea for a homemade gift.

1 (3.3-oz) jar sugar-free iced tea   2 (1.8-oz) pkg. sugar-free orange
  mix with lemon   breakfast drink mix
1 tbsp. plus 1 tsp. ground   2 tsp. ground cloves
  cinnamon

Combine all ingredients. Use an airtight container, or package into three 1-cup gift packages. (Gift tag instructions: "To serve hot, stir $1^1/_2$ teaspoons of mixture into 1 cup hot water.")

Nutritional Information per one-cup serving: 3 calories.

Apricot Spread

Note: Great idea for a homemade gift.

1 cup dried apricots
1 cup unsweetened apple juice

Combine apricots and apple juice in a small saucepan; bring to boil over medium-high heat. Reduce heat to low; cover and simmer 20 minutes, stirring occasionally. Remove from heat and allow to cool slightly. Pour cooled mixture into blender or food processor and blend until smooth. Finish cooling to room temperature and refrigerate in airtight container or jar with tight-fitting lid up to 3 months. Serves 15.

Nutritional Information: 27 calories; trace fat (2% calories from fat); trace protein; 7g carbohydrate; 1g dietary fiber; 0mg cholesterol; 1mg sodium.

Cappuccino Mix

Note: Keep a container of this mix handy for entertaining or for when you curl up in your favorite chair to study your Bible!

1¹/₂ cups powdered fat-free nondairy creamer	²/₃ cup decaffeinated instant coffee
¹/₂ cup cocoa powder	1 tsp. ground cinnamon
³/₄ cup sugar substitute	¹/₄ tsp. ground nutmeg

Combine all ingredients; mix well and store in airtight container. When ready to use, add 3 level tablespoons of mix to 1¹/₂ cups boiling water. Stir and enjoy! Serves 16.

Nutritional Information: 40 calories; trace fat (9% calories from fat); 1g protein; 9g carbohydrate; 1g dietary fiber; 0mg cholesterol; 19mg sodium.

Creamy Cucumber Dip

1 cucumber	3 tbsp. chile sauce
¹/₂ bunch medium-sized radishes	¹/₄ tsp. minced garlic

$^1/_2$ green bell pepper

$^1/_2$ cup chopped green onions,
tops included

1 cup fat-free sour cream

$^1/_2$ cup fat-free Miracle Whip

Dash cayenne pepper

$^1/_2$ tsp. crushed dried dill seed

1 tsp. crushed dried parsley

$^1/_2$ tsp. salt

Grate cucumber using food processor's grating blade. Press with paper towel to remove excess liquid. Replace grating blade with cutting blade, add radishes, bell pepper and onions to cucumber. Mix quickly, but do not liquefy. Drain excess liquid. Add sour cream, Miracle Whip, chile sauce, garlic, cayenne pepper, dill weed, parsley and salt. Mix well by hand, chill and serve with fresh vegetables, baked chips or crackers. Serves 16.

Nutritional Information: 36 calories; 2g fat (47% calories from fat); 1g protein; 4g carbohydrate; trace dietary fiber; 4mg cholesterol; 126mg sodium.

Spinach Dip

1 (10-oz.) pkg. frozen chopped
spinach, thawed and well drained

1 cup fat-free Miracle Whip

1 cup fat-free sour cream

1 tbsp. minced onion

1 envelope vegetable soup mix

Combine all ingredients in a small bowl. Refrigerate overnight to allow flavors to blend. Serve with *Toasted Pita Chips*. Serves 6.

Nutritional Information: 44 calories; trace fat (4% calories from fat); 5g protein; 7g carbohydrate; 2g dietary fiber; 4mg cholesterol; 85mg sodium.

Toasted Pita Chips

Note: These are great with dips, in soups and with lunches. For more fiber, use whole-wheat pita bread.

2 (6-inch) pita bread pockets
1/4 tsp. garlic salt

Butter-flavored nonstick
cooking spray

Preheat oven to 325° F. Split each pita pocket in half with a sharp knife; cut each half into 6 triangles (24 total). Arrange triangles in single layers on cookie sheets, coat with cooking spray and sprinkle lightly with garlic salt. Bake for 8 minutes or until chips are lightly browned and very crisp. Store in airtight container until ready to serve. Serves 4.

Nutritional Information: 83 calories; trace fat (4% calories from fat); 3g protein; 17g carbohydrate; 1g dietary fiber; 0mg cholesterol; 289mg sodium.

Ranch-Style Breaded Chicken

4 boneless, skinless chicken breasts
1 (1-oz.) pkg. Ranch dressing mix
4 oz. fat-free cheddar
  cheese, shredded

2 egg whites
Nonstick cooking spray
20 fat-free saltine
  crackers, crushed

Preheat oven to 350° F. Place cheese, Ranch dressing mix and cracker crumbs each in their own shallow dish or plate; set aside. Slightly beat egg whites in small bowl. One at a time, dip chicken breasts in egg whites; then roll in cheese, dressing mix and cracker crumbs. Place coated chicken breast on baking sheet coated with cooking spray; repeat with remaining breasts. Bake 35 to 40 minutes. Serves 4.

Nutritional Information: 292 calories; 2g fat (6% calories from fat); 3g monounsaturated fat; 40g protein; 26g carbohydrate; 1g dietary fiber; 71mg cholesterol; 974mg sodium.

Slow "Souper" Chile Chicken

8 boneless, skinless chicken
  breast halves, diced
1 (14.5-oz.) can diced tomatoes

1 (11-oz.) can corn, drained
1 (10.7-oz.) can low-fat cream
  of chicken soup

3 (4.5-oz.) cans chopped
  green chilies
1 (15.5-oz.) can pinto beans,
  rinsed and drained
1 (14.5-oz.) can tomatoes
  with green chilies

1 large onion, chopped
1 tsp. chicken bouillon
1 tsp. minced garlic
$1/4$ tsp. cumin
$1/4$ tsp. oregano

Place all ingredients in order into slow cooker set to Low heat. Cover and cook 7 to 8 hours (or 4 hours on High). Top each 1 cup serving of soup with 1 tbsp. sour cream, 1 tbsp. cheese, 2 broken tortilla chips, and chopped green onion and cilantro to taste. Serves 12.

Nutritional Information: 315 calories; 7g fat (19% calories from fat); 3g saturated fat; 6g monounsaturated fat; 2g polyunsaturated fat; 44g protein; 19g carbohydrate; 5g dietary fiber; 101mg cholesterol; 451mg sodium.

Oven Roasted Vegetables

1 cup fresh cauliflower
  pieces (bite-sized)
1 cup fresh broccoli
  pieces (bite-sized)
$1/2$ cup sliced celery,
  cut into bite-sized pieces
$1/3$ cup chopped red onion
1 cup mushroom caps

$1/4$ cup sliced carrots
$1/3$ cup cherry-tomato halves
1 tbsp. lemon juice
$1/4$ tsp. dried dill weed
2 tbsp. low-fat Ranch dressing
Butter-flavored nonstick
  cooking spray

Preheat oven to 400° F. In large bowl, combine cauliflower, broccoli, celery, onion, carrots, mushrooms and tomatoes, toss to mix. Arrange vegetables on baking pan coated with cooking spray. Spray vegetables lightly with cooking spray; bake 20 minutes or until tender. While vegetables are cooking, use same bowl to combine lemon juice, dill weed and dressing. Mix well and set aside. Remove vegetables from oven, drain and return to bowl. Toss to coat. Serve hot. Serves 4.

Nutritional Information: 30 calories; trace fat (6% calories from fat); 2g protein; 6g carbohydrate; 2g dietary fiber; 0mg cholesterol; 31mg sodium.

Brunch Casserole

4 slices whole-wheat bread,
   crusts removed
2 oz. ground low-fat
   turkey sausage
1/2 cup chopped mushrooms
1 tsp. chopped onion
3 eggs, beaten

1 cup nonfat milk
1/4 tsp. salt
1/8 tsp. black pepper
1/8 tsp. granulated garlic
2 oz. low-fat cheddar
   cheese, shredded

Line bottom of 9 x 9 casserole dish with bread. Sauté sausage in nonstick skillet until cooked through. Remove sausage and sauté mushrooms and onions until tender. Crumble sausage and combine with mushrooms and onion; sprinkle mixture on top of bread. Combine eggs, milk, salt, pepper and garlic, mix well and pour over sausage. Sprinkle with cheese, cover and refrigerate overnight. Set out for 15 minutes prior to baking. Bake at 350° F for 40 to 45 minutes. Serves 4.

Nutritional Information: 199 calories; 7g fat (33% calories from fat); 3g saturated fat; 2g monounsaturated fat; 1g polyunsaturated fat; 16g protein; 17g carbohydrate; 2g dietary fiber; 175mg cholesterol; 537mg sodium.

Bread Pudding Breakfast Dish

3 egg whites
1/2 cup nonfat milk
1 tsp. vanilla extract
2 tsp. sugar substitute

1 slice Texas-style bread,
   broken into chunks
1 tsp. raisins

In a microwave-safe bowl, combine egg whites, milk, vanilla and sugar substitute; fold in bread chunks and raisins, then microwave on High for 3 minutes. Serves 1.

Nutritional Information: 199 calories; 1g fat (6% calories from fat); 17g protein; 27g carbohydrate; 1g dietary fiber; 2mg cholesterol; 378mg sodium.

Chocolate Banana Cream Pie

8 graham crackers, divided into 16 pieces
1 (1.5-oz.) box sugar-free, white-chocolate-flavored nonfat instant pudding
3¹/₂ cups nonfat milk
1 (1.5-oz.) box sugar-free, chocolate-flavored nonfat instant pudding
2 bananas, sliced
3 cups fat-free whipped topping

Line a pie plate (or oblong baking dish) with graham-cracker pieces; set aside. Prepare puddings in separate bowls, mixing each with 1³/₄ cups milk and whipping until set. Pour white-chocolate pudding over top of graham crackers; layer with banana slices and top with chocolate pudding. Refrigerate 2 hours or until set. Top with whipped topping prior to serving. Serves 8.

Nutritional Information: 121 calories; 1g fat (10% calories from fat); 4g protein; 17g carbohydrate; 1g dietary fiber; 2mg cholesterol; 98mg sodium.

Peach Pudding Cake

Note: This is delicious served warm with ¹/₄ cup sugar-free vanilla-flavored nonfat ice cream.

2 cups fresh or frozen peaches
1 tsp. ground cinnamon
¹/₂ cup nonfat milk
3 tbsp. fat-free liquid margarine

1 tsp. lemon juice

1 cup all-purpose flour

1¹/₂ cups sugar substitute

1 tsp. baking powder

1 tbsp. cornstarch

1 cup boiling water

Nonstick cooking spray

Preheat oven to 350° F. In small bowl, toss peaches with cinnamon and lemon juice, then arrange in 8 x 8 baking dish coated with cooking spray and set aside. In medium bowl, combine flour, ³/₄ cup sugar substitute and baking powder, mix well. Stir in milk and margarine; spoon evenly over fruit in baking dish. In small bowl, combine remaining sugar substitute with cornstarch; sprinkle over milk-margarine mixture. Slowly pour boiling water over top; bake 45 to 50 minutes or until toothpick comes out clean. Serves 6.

Nutritional Information: 289 calories; trace fat (1% calories from fat); 3g protein; 61g carbohydrate; 2g dietary fiber; trace cholesterol; 240mg sodium.

Frozen Snicker Pie

1 low-fat graham cracker crust

1 cup Cool Whip Lite

12 oz. sugar-free vanilla-flavored
  nonfat frozen yogurt
  (or fat-free ice cream)

1 (1.5-oz.) box sugar-free chocolate-
  flavored instant pudding

3 tbsp. chunky peanut butter

Press graham-cracker crumbs into an 8 x 8 baking dish; set aside. In large bowl, combine frozen yogurt, whipped topping, peanut butter and pudding mix; stir well and pour into pan, being careful not to disturb the crumbs. Freeze 2 hours or until firm. Let thaw 10 minutes before serving. Serves 8.

Nutritional Information: 122 calories; 4g fat (32% calories from fat); 1g saturated fat; 1g monounsaturated fat; 1g polyunsaturated fat; 4g protein; 15g carbohydrate; trace dietary fiber; 0mg cholesterol; 74mg sodium.

Double Layer Chocolate Pie

1¹/₂ cups plus 1 tbsp.
  cold skim milk
2 (1.5-oz.) boxes chocolate-
  flavored sugar-free
  instant pudding
1 pkg. sugar substitute

4 oz. fat-free cream
  cheese, softened
4 oz. Cool Whip Lite
1 low-fat graham
  cracker crust

Pour 1¹/₂ cups milk into medium bowl; add pudding mix. Beat with an electric mixer for one minute (mixture will be very thick). Spread mixture evenly into piecrust. Beat cream cheese, sweetener and 1 tbsp. milk with mixer until smooth. Fold in Cool Whip on Low speed. Spread over chocolate mixture. Cover and chill at least 3 hours before serving. Serves 8.

Nutritional Information: 204 calories; 8g fat (39% calories from fat); 1g saturated fat; 5g protein; 23g carbohydrate; trace dietary fiber; 2mg cholesterol; 272mg sodium.

Chex Party Mix

¹/₄ cup light margarine
1 tbsp. Worcestershire sauce
¹/₄ tsp. celery salt
¹/₄ tsp. seasoned salt
¹/₄ tsp. garlic salt
2 cups Chex rice cereal
2 cups Chex wheat cereal

2 cups Chex corn cereal
1 cup plain Cheerios
1 cup pretzel sticks or
  oyster crackers
Butter-flavored nonstick
  cooking spray

Preheat oven to 325° F. In small saucepan, heat margarine and seasonings, stirring until combined. In a very large bowl, toss remaining ingredients with margarine mixture. Spread cereal mixture evenly over an 11 x 7 pan sprayed with nonstick cooking spray. Bake 20 minutes, stirring occasionally. Serve immediately or store in an airtight container. Serves 16.

Nutritional Information per half-cup serving: 31 calories; 2g fat (43% calories from fat); 1g monounsaturated fat; 1g polyunsaturated fat; 1g protein; 4g carbohydrate; trace dietary fiber; 0mg cholesterol; 184mg sodium.

New Year's Day Menus and Recipes

Note: Recipes for items *italicized in bold* are included below.

MENUS

Breakfast

1 slice whole-wheat bread

1/2 tbsp. light margarine

3 egg whites, scrambled

1/2 grapefruit

1 cup nonfat milk

Nutritional Information: 267 calories; 5g fat (15% calories from fat); 22g protein; 35g carbohydrate; 3g dietary fiber; 4mg cholesterol; 507mg sodium.

New Year's Day Meal

1 serving *Pasta E Fagioli*

1 piece *Blue Ribbon Cornbread*

1 serving *Creamy Fruit Salad*

Nutritional Information: 431 calories; 9g fat (20% calories from fat); 3g saturated fat; 3g monounsaturated fat; 1g polyunsaturated fat; 17g protein; 74g carbohydrate; 9g dietary fiber; 39mg cholesterol; 531mg sodium.

Dinner

(May be used for lunch or dinner.)

1 *French-Dip Roast Beef Sandwich*

1 cup strawberries

1 cup broccoli florets served with

2 tbsp. low-fat Ranch dressing

Nutritional Information: 369 calories; 12g fat (30% calories from fat); 4g saturated fat; 4g monounsaturated fat; 1g polyunsaturated fat; 22g protein; 45g carbohydrate; 8g dietary fiber; 33mg cholesterol; 1,034mg sodium.

Healthy Snack Options

1 cup nonfat dairy yogurt with 1/2 banana

3 cups light microwave popcorn

1 *Tortilla Roll Up*

RECIPES

Pasta E Fagioli

1 lb. lean ground beef

2 tsp. olive oil

2 large onions, chopped

2 cups diced carrots

2 cups diced celery

3 cups diced zucchini

6 cups water

1/2 cup granulated beef bouillon

2 tsp. dried oregano

1 tsp. black pepper

3 tbsp. parsley

2 tsp. hot pepper sauce

6 cups chunky pasta sauce

1 (15-oz.) can red kidney beans,
   drained and rinsed

1 (19-oz.) can white kidney beans,
   drained and rinsed

2 cups cooked macaroni or
   small pasta shells

In a preheated soup pot, brown ground beef with olive oil over medium-high heat, stirring constantly to break up. Add onion, carrots, celery and zucchini; sauté 10 minutes more, then reduce heat to simmer. Dissolve beef bouillon in small bowl with 1 cup hot water; stir in oregano, black pepper, parsley and hot pepper sauce. Add mixture to beef mixture, then stir in pasta sauce and simmer 10 minutes. Stir in remaining 5 cups water (or enough to reach desired consistency) and simmer 30 minutes more, stirring occasionally. Add beans and pasta just prior to serving. Serves 16.

Nutritional Information: 205 calories; 7g fat (30% calories from fat); 3g saturated fat; 3g monounsaturated fat; 1g polyunsaturated fat; 12g protein; 24g carbohydrate; 5g dietary fiber; 21mg cholesterol; 104mg sodium.

Blue Ribbon Cornbread

1 cup cornmeal

1 cup flour

$^1/_2$ tsp. salt

1 tbsp. baking powder

1 egg

1 cup nonfat milk

4 oz. sugar-free vanilla-
flavored nonfat yogurt

Nonstick cooking spray

Preheat oven to 425° F. In large bowl, combine cornmeal, flour, salt and baking powder; mix well. Add egg, milk and yogurt; stir to combine and pour into 9 x 9 baking dish coated with cooking spray. Bake 20 minutes or until lightly browned. Serves 12.

Nutritional Information: 125 calories; 1g fat (5% calories from fat); 3g protein; 26g carbohydrate; 1g dietary fiber; 18mg cholesterol; 409mg sodium.

Creamy Fruit Salad

1 (15-oz.) can chunky mixed
fruit in juice, drained

2 medium bananas, sliced

1 cup sliced strawberries

$^1/_2$ cup sugar-free lemon-
flavored low-fat yogurt

$^1/_2$ cup fat-free whipped topping

Combine mixed fruit, bananas and strawberries in medium bowl. Gently fold in yogurt and whipped topping until fruit is coated. Refrigerate until ready to serve. Serves 4.

Nutritional Information: 101 calories; 1g fat (4% calories from fat); 2g protein; 24g carbohydrate; 3g dietary fiber; trace cholesterol; 18mg sodium.

French-Dip Roast Beef Sandwich

1 (4-oz.) loaf French bread

1 cup low-sodium beef broth,
heated

4 oz. cooked, lean, boneless roast
beef, thinly sliced

Cut bread loaf in half horizontally; then cut pieces in half vertically to make 4 pieces. Place 2 bread pieces, cut side up, on each of 2 plates. Top each with 1 ounce of roast beef and $1/4$ cup broth. Cover each plate with plastic wrap; microwave for 30 to 45 seconds until hot. Serves 2.

Nutritional Information: 303 calories; 11g fat (32% calories from fat); 4g saturated fat; 4g monounsaturated fat; 1g polyunsaturated fat; 19g protein; 31g carbohydrate; 2g dietary fiber; 33mg cholesterol; 1,013mg sodium.

Tortilla Roll-Ups

6 (6-inch) low-fat flour tortillas $1/4$ cup chunky salsa
8 oz. fat-free cream cheese, softened

Mix cream cheese and salsa in small bowl; stir well to combine. Cover one side of each tortilla with an equal amount of cream-cheese blend; roll tortillas and place on serving platter. Cover with plastic wrap and refrigerate at least 1 hour. Slice into 1-inch pieces just prior to serving. Serves 6.

Nutritional Information: 169 calories; 2g fat (12% calories from fat); 6g protein; 29g carbohydrate; 3g dietary fiber; 3mg cholesterol; 583mg sodium.

Member Survey

Please answer the following questions to help your leader plan your First Place 4 Health meetings so that your needs might be met in this session. Give this form to your leader at the first group meeting.

Name _____ Birth date _____

Please list those who live in your household.

Name	Relationship	Age
_____	_____	_____
_____	_____	_____
_____	_____	_____
_____	_____	_____

What church do you attend? _____

Are you interested in receiving more information about our church?

❒ Yes   ❒ No

Occupation _____

What talent or area of expertise would you be willing to share with our class?

_____

Why did you join First Place 4 Health?

_____

With notice, would you be willing to lead a Bible study discussion one week?

❒ Yes   ❒ No

Are you comfortable praying out loud? _____

If the assistant leader were absent, would you be willing to assist in weighing in members and possibly evaluating the Live It Trackers?

❒ Yes   ❒ No

Any other comments:

_____

_____

Personal Weight and Measurement Record

Week	Weight	+ or -	Goal this Session	Pounds to goal
1				
2				
3				
4				
5				
6				

Beginning Measurements

Waist _____ Hips _____ Thighs _____ Chest _____

Ending Measurements

Waist _____ Hips _____ Thighs _____ Chest _____

First Place 4 Health
Prayer Partner

LIGHT & HEALTHY
HOLIDAYS
Week
1

Give thanks in all circumstances
for this is God's will for you in Christ Jesus.

1 THESSALONIANS 5:18

Date: _____

Name: _____

Home Phone: (_____) _____

Work Phone: (_____) _____

Email: _____

Personal Prayer Concerns:

_____

_____

_____

_____

_____

_____

_____

This form is for prayer requests that are personal to you and your journey in First Place 4 Health. Please complete this form and have it ready to turn in when you arrive at your group meeting.

First Place 4 Health
Prayer Partner

4 first place
health

Give thanks to the Lord, for He is good;
His love endures forever.

1 CHRONICLES 16:34

Date: _____

Name: _____

Home Phone: (_____) _____

Work Phone: (_____) _____

Email: _____

Personal Prayer Concerns:

_____

_____

_____

_____

_____

_____

_____

This form is for prayer requests that are personal to you and your journey in First Place 4 Health. Please complete this form and have it ready to turn in when you arrive at your group meeting.

First Place 4 Health
Prayer Partner

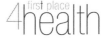

But the angel said to them, "Do not be afraid. I bring you good news of great joy
that will be for all the people. Today in the town of David a Savior
has been born to you; He is Christ the Lord."

Luke 2:10-11

Date: _____

Name: _____

Home Phone: (_____) _____

Work Phone: (_____) _____

Email: _____

Personal Prayer Concerns:

_____

_____

_____

_____

_____

_____

_____

This form is for prayer requests that are personal to you and your journey in First Place 4 Health. Please complete this form and have it ready to turn in when you arrive at your group meeting.

First Place 4 Health
Prayer Partner

LIGHT & HEALTHY
HOLIDAYS
Week
4

*After Jesus was born in Bethlehem in Judea, during the time of King Herod, Magi
from the east came to Jerusalem and asked, "Where is the one who has been born
king of the Jews? We saw his star in the east and have come to worship Him."*

MATTHEW 2:1-2

Date: _____

Name: _____

Home Phone: (_____) _____

Work Phone: (_____) _____

Email: _____

Personal Prayer Concerns:

_____

_____

_____

_____

_____

_____

_____

This form is for prayer requests that are personal to you and your journey in First Place 4 Health. Please complete this
form and have it ready to turn in when you arrive at your group meeting.

First Place 4 Health
Prayer Partner

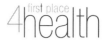

You were taught, with regard to your former way of life, to put off your old self, which is being corrupted by its deceitful desires; to be made new in the attitudes of your minds; and to put on the new self, created to be like God in true righteousness and holiness.

EPHESIANS 4:22-24

Date: _____

Name: _____

Home Phone: (_____) _____

Work Phone: (_____) _____

Email: _____

Personal Prayer Concerns:

_____

_____

_____

_____

_____

_____

_____

This form is for prayer requests that are personal to you and your journey in First Place 4 Health. Please complete this form and have it ready to turn in when you arrive at your group meeting.

First Place 4 Health
Prayer Partner

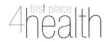

LIGHT & HEALTHY
HOLIDAYS
Week
6

*I will give you a new heart and put a new spirit in you; I will remove from
you your heart of stone and give you a heart of flesh.*

EZEKIEL 36:26

Date: _____

Name: _____

Home Phone: (_____) _____

Work Phone: (_____) _____

Email: _____

Personal Prayer Concerns:

_____

_____

_____

_____

_____

_____

_____

This form is for prayer requests that are personal to you and your journey in First Place 4 Health. Please complete this form and have it ready to turn in when you arrive at your group meeting.

Live It Tracker

Name: _____   My week at a glance: ❑ Great ❑ So-so ❑ Not so great

Date: _____ Week #: _____ Calorie Range: _____   My food goal for next week: _____

Activity Level: None, < 30 min/day, 30-60 min/day, 60+ min/day   My activity goal for next week: _____

Scripture Memory Verse: _____

RECOMMENDED DAILY AMOUNT OF FOOD FROM EACH GROUP

Group	Daily Calories							
	1300-1400	1500-1600	1700-1800	1900-2000	2100-2200	2300-2400	2500-2600	2700-2800
Fruits	1.5-2 c.	1.5-2 c.	1.5-2 c.	2-2.5 c.	2-2.5 c.	2.5-3.5 c.	3.5-4.5 c.	3.5-4.5 c.
Vegetables	1.5-2 c.	2-2.5 c.	2.5-3 c.	2.5-3 c.	3-3.5 c.	3.5-4.5 c.	4.5-5 c.	4.5-5 c.
Grains	5 oz-eq.	5-6 oz-eq.	6-7 oz-eq.	6-7 oz-eq.	7-8 oz-eq.	8-9 oz-eq.	9-10 oz-eq.	10-11 oz-eq.
Meat & Beans	4 oz-eq.	5 oz-eq.	5-5.5 oz-eq.	5.5-6.5 oz-eq.	6.5-7 oz-eq.	7-7.5 oz-eq.	7-7.5 oz-eq.	7.5-8 oz-eq.
Milk	2-3 c.	3 c.	3 c.	3 c.	3 c.	3 c.	3 c.	3 c.
Healthy Oils	4 tsp.	5 tsp.	5 tsp.	6 tsp.	6 tsp.	7 tsp.	8 tsp.	8 tsp.

Day One

FOOD CHOICES

Breakfast: _____   Lunch: _____

Dinner: _____   Snacks: _____

Group	Fruits	Vegetables	Grains	Meat & Beans	Milk	Oils
Goal Amount						
Estimate Your Total						
Increase ⇧ or Decrease ⇩ ?						

PHYSICAL ACTIVITY   **SPIRITUAL ACTIVITY**

Description: _____   Description: _____

Steps/Miles/Minutes: _____

Day Two

FOOD CHOICES

Breakfast: _____   Lunch: _____

Dinner: _____   Snacks: _____

Group	Fruits	Vegetables	Grains	Meat & Beans	Milk	Oils
Goal Amount						
Estimate Your Total						
Increase ⇧ or Decrease ⇩ ?						

PHYSICAL ACTIVITY   **SPIRITUAL ACTIVITY**

Description: _____   Description: _____

Steps/Miles/Minutes: _____

Day Three

FOOD CHOICES

Breakfast: _____   Lunch: _____

Dinner: _____   Snacks: _____

Group	Fruits	Vegetables	Grains	Meat & Beans	Milk	Oils
Goal Amount						
Estimate Your Total						
Increase ⇧ or Decrease ⇩ ?						

PHYSICAL ACTIVITY   **SPIRITUAL ACTIVITY**

Description: _____   Description: _____

Steps/Miles/Minutes: _____

FOOD CHOICES

Day Four

Breakfast: _____ Lunch: _____

Dinner: _____ Snacks: _____

Group	Fruits	Vegetables	Grains	Meat & Beans	Milk	Oils
Goal Amount						
Estimate Your Total						
Increase ⇧ or Decrease ⇩ ?						

PHYSICAL ACTIVITY

Description: _____

Steps/Miles/Minutes: _____

SPIRITUAL ACTIVITY

Description: _____

_____

FOOD CHOICES

Day Five

Breakfast: _____ Lunch: _____

Dinner: _____ Snacks: _____

Group	Fruits	Vegetables	Grains	Meat & Beans	Milk	Oils
Goal Amount						
Estimate Your Total						
Increase ⇧ or Decrease ⇩ ?						

PHYSICAL ACTIVITY

Description: _____

Steps/Miles/Minutes: _____

SPIRITUAL ACTIVITY

Description: _____

_____

FOOD CHOICES

Day Six

Breakfast: _____ Lunch: _____

Dinner: _____ Snacks: _____

Group	Fruits	Vegetables	Grains	Meat & Beans	Milk	Oils
Goal Amount						
Estimate Your Total						
Increase ⇧ or Decrease ⇩ ?						

PHYSICAL ACTIVITY

Description: _____

Steps/Miles/Minutes: _____

SPIRITUAL ACTIVITY

Description: _____

_____

FOOD CHOICES

Day Seven

Breakfast: _____ Lunch: _____

Dinner: _____ Snacks: _____

Group	Fruits	Vegetables	Grains	Meat & Beans	Milk	Oils
Goal Amount						
Estimate Your Total						
Increase ⇧ or Decrease ⇩ ?						

PHYSICAL ACTIVITY

Description: _____

Steps/Miles/Minutes: _____

SPIRITUAL ACTIVITY

Description: _____

_____

Live It Tracker

Name: _____   My week at a glance: ☐ Great ☐ So-so ☐ Not so great

Date: _____ Week #: _____ Calorie Range: _____   My food goal for next week: _____

Activity Level: None, < 30 min/day, 30-60 min/day, 60+ min/day   My activity goal for next week: _____

Scripture Memory Verse: _____

RECOMMENDED DAILY AMOUNT OF FOOD FROM EACH GROUP

Group	Daily Calories							
	1300-1400	1500-1600	1700-1800	1900-2000	2100-2200	2300-2400	2500-2600	2700-2800
Fruits	1.5-2 c.	1.5-2 c.	1.5-2 c.	2-2.5 c.	2-2.5 c.	2.5-3.5 c.	3.5-4.5 c.	3.5-4.5 c.
Vegetables	1.5-2 c.	2-2.5 c.	2.5-3 c.	2.5-3 c.	3-3.5 c.	3.5-4.5 c.	4.5-5 c.	4.5-5 c.
Grains	5 oz-eq.	5-6 oz-eq.	6-7 oz-eq.	6-7 oz-eq.	7-8 oz-eq.	8-9 oz-eq.	9-10 oz-eq.	10-11 oz-eq.
Meat & Beans	4 oz-eq.	5 oz-eq.	5-5.5 oz-eq.	5.5-6.5 oz-eq.	6.5-7 oz-eq.	7-7.5 oz-eq.	7-7.5 oz-eq.	7.5-8 oz-eq.
Milk	2-3 c.	3 c.	3 c.	3 c.	3 c.	3 c.	3 c.	3 c.
Healthy Oils	4 tsp.	5 tsp.	5 tsp.	6 tsp.	6 tsp.	7 tsp	8 tsp.	8 tsp.

Day One

FOOD CHOICES

Breakfast: _____   Lunch: _____

Dinner: _____   Snacks: _____

Group	Fruits	Vegetables	Grains	Meat & Beans	Milk	Oils
Goal Amount						
Estimate Your Total						
Increase ⇧ or Decrease ⇩ ?						

PHYSICAL ACTIVITY

Description: _____

Steps/Miles/Minutes: _____

SPIRITUAL ACTIVITY

Description: _____

Day Two

FOOD CHOICES

Breakfast: _____   Lunch: _____

Dinner: _____   Snacks: _____

Group	Fruits	Vegetables	Grains	Meat & Beans	Milk	Oils
Goal Amount						
Estimate Your Total						
Increase ⇧ or Decrease ⇩ ?						

PHYSICAL ACTIVITY

Description: _____

Steps/Miles/Minutes: _____

SPIRITUAL ACTIVITY

Description: _____

Day Three

FOOD CHOICES

Breakfast: _____   Lunch: _____

Dinner: _____   Snacks: _____

Group	Fruits	Vegetables	Grains	Meat & Beans	Milk	Oils
Goal Amount						
Estimate Your Total						
Increase ⇧ or Decrease ⇩ ?						

PHYSICAL ACTIVITY

Description: _____

Steps/Miles/Minutes: _____

SPIRITUAL ACTIVITY

Description: _____

Day Four

FOOD CHOICES

Breakfast: _____ Lunch: _____

Dinner: _____ Snacks: _____

Group	Fruits	Vegetables	Grains	Meat & Beans	Milk	Oils
Goal Amount						
Estimate Your Total						
Increase ⇧ or Decrease ⇩ ?						

PHYSICAL ACTIVITY

Description: _____

Steps/Miles/Minutes: _____

SPIRITUAL ACTIVITY

Description: _____

_____

Day Five

FOOD CHOICES

Breakfast: _____ Lunch: _____

Dinner: _____ Snacks: _____

Group	Fruits	Vegetables	Grains	Meat & Beans	Milk	Oils
Goal Amount						
Estimate Your Total						
Increase ⇧ or Decrease ⇩ ?						

PHYSICAL ACTIVITY

Description: _____

Steps/Miles/Minutes: _____

SPIRITUAL ACTIVITY

Description: _____

_____

Day Six

FOOD CHOICES

Breakfast: _____ Lunch: _____

Dinner: _____ Snacks: _____

Group	Fruits	Vegetables	Grains	Meat & Beans	Milk	Oils
Goal Amount						
Estimate Your Total						
Increase ⇧ or Decrease ⇩ ?						

PHYSICAL ACTIVITY

Description: _____

Steps/Miles/Minutes: _____

SPIRITUAL ACTIVITY

Description: _____

_____

Day Seven

FOOD CHOICES

Breakfast: _____ Lunch: _____

Dinner: _____ Snacks: _____

Group	Fruits	Vegetables	Grains	Meat & Beans	Milk	Oils
Goal Amount						
Estimate Your Total						
Increase ⇧ or Decrease ⇩ ?						

PHYSICAL ACTIVITY

Description: _____

Steps/Miles/Minutes: _____

SPIRITUAL ACTIVITY

Description: _____

_____

Live It Tracker

Name: _____   My week at a glance: ❏ Great ❏ So-so ❏ Not so great

Date: _____ Week #: _____ Calorie Range: _____   My food goal for next week: _____

Activity Level: None, < 30 min/day, 30-60 min/day, 60+ min/day   My activity goal for next week: _____

Scripture Memory Verse: _____

_____

RECOMMENDED DAILY AMOUNT OF FOOD FROM EACH GROUP

Group	Daily Calories							
	1300-1400	1500-1600	1700-1800	1900-2000	2100-2200	2300-2400	2500-2600	2700-2800
Fruits	1.5-2 c.	1.5-2 c.	1.5-2 c.	2-2.5 c.	2-2.5 c.	2.5-3.5 c.	3.5-4.5 c.	3.5-4.5 c.
Vegetables	1.5-2 c.	2-2.5 c.	2.5-3 c.	2.5-3 c.	3-3.5 c.	3.5-4.5 c.	4.5-5 c.	4.5-5 c.
Grains	5 oz-eq.	5-6 oz-eq.	6-7 oz-eq.	6-7 oz-eq.	7-8 oz-eq.	8-9 oz-eq.	9-10 oz-eq.	10-11 oz-eq.
Meat & Beans	4 oz-eq.	5 oz-eq.	5-5.5 oz-eq.	5.5-6.5 oz-eq.	6.5-7 oz-eq.	7-7.5 oz-eq.	7-7.5 oz-eq.	7.5-8 oz-eq.
Milk	2-3 c.	3 c.	3 c.	3 c.	3 c.	3 c.	3 c.	3 c.
Healthy Oils	4 tsp.	5 tsp.	5 tsp.	6 tsp.	6 tsp.	7 tsp.	8 tsp.	8 tsp.

Day One

FOOD CHOICES

Breakfast: _____   Lunch: _____

Dinner: _____   Snacks: _____

Group	Fruits	Vegetables	Grains	Meat & Beans	Milk	Oils
Goal Amount						
Estimate Your Total						
Increase ⇧ or Decrease ⇩ ?						

PHYSICAL ACTIVITY

Description: _____

Steps/Miles/Minutes: _____

SPIRITUAL ACTIVITY

Description: _____

_____

Day Two

FOOD CHOICES

Breakfast: _____   Lunch: _____

Dinner: _____   Snacks: _____

Group	Fruits	Vegetables	Grains	Meat & Beans	Milk	Oils
Goal Amount						
Estimate Your Total						
Increase ⇧ or Decrease ⇩ ?						

PHYSICAL ACTIVITY

Description: _____

Steps/Miles/Minutes: _____

SPIRITUAL ACTIVITY

Description: _____

_____

Day Three

FOOD CHOICES

Breakfast: _____   Lunch: _____

Dinner: _____   Snacks: _____

Group	Fruits	Vegetables	Grains	Meat & Beans	Milk	Oils
Goal Amount						
Estimate Your Total						
Increase ⇧ or Decrease ⇩ ?						

PHYSICAL ACTIVITY

Description: _____

Steps/Miles/Minutes: _____

SPIRITUAL ACTIVITY

Description: _____

_____

Day Four

FOOD CHOICES

Breakfast: _____ Lunch: _____

Dinner: _____ Snacks: _____

Group	Fruits	Vegetables	Grains	Meat & Beans	Milk	Oils
Goal Amount						
Estimate Your Total						
Increase ⇧ or Decrease ⇩ ?						

PHYSICAL ACTIVITY

Description: _____

Steps/Miles/Minutes: _____

SPIRITUAL ACTIVITY

Description: _____

_____

Day Five

FOOD CHOICES

Breakfast: _____ Lunch: _____

Dinner: _____ Snacks: _____

Group	Fruits	Vegetables	Grains	Meat & Beans	Milk	Oils
Goal Amount						
Estimate Your Total						
Increase ⇧ or Decrease ⇩ ?						

PHYSICAL ACTIVITY

Description: _____

Steps/Miles/Minutes: _____

SPIRITUAL ACTIVITY

Description: _____

_____

Day Six

FOOD CHOICES

Breakfast: _____ Lunch: _____

Dinner: _____ Snacks: _____

Group	Fruits	Vegetables	Grains	Meat & Beans	Milk	Oils
Goal Amount						
Estimate Your Total						
Increase ⇧ or Decrease ⇩ ?						

PHYSICAL ACTIVITY

Description: _____

Steps/Miles/Minutes: _____

SPIRITUAL ACTIVITY

Description: _____

_____

Day Seven

FOOD CHOICES

Breakfast: _____ Lunch: _____

Dinner: _____ Snacks: _____

Group	Fruits	Vegetables	Grains	Meat & Beans	Milk	Oils
Goal Amount						
Estimate Your Total						
Increase ⇧ or Decrease ⇩ ?						

PHYSICAL ACTIVITY

Description: _____

Steps/Miles/Minutes: _____

SPIRITUAL ACTIVITY

Description: _____

_____

Live It Tracker

Name: _____   My week at a glance: ❏ Great ❏ So-so ❏ Not so great

Date: _____ Week #: _____ Calorie Range: _____   My food goal for next week: _____

Activity Level: None, < 30 min/day, 30-60 min/day, 60+ min/day   My activity goal for next week: _____

Scripture Memory Verse: _____

RECOMMENDED DAILY AMOUNT OF FOOD FROM EACH GROUP

Group	Daily Calories							
	1300-1400	1500-1600	1700-1800	1900-2000	2100-2200	2300-2400	2500-2600	2700-2800
Fruits	1.5-2 c.	1.5-2 c.	1.5-2 c.	2-2.5 c.	2-2.5 c.	2.5-3.5 c.	3.5-4.5 c.	3.5-4.5 c.
Vegetables	1.5-2 c.	2-2.5 c.	2.5-3 c.	2.5-3 c.	3-3.5 c.	3.5-4.5 c.	4.5-5 c.	4.5-5 c.
Grains	5 oz-eq.	5-6 oz-eq.	6-7 oz-eq.	6-7 oz-eq.	7-8 oz-eq.	8-9 oz-eq.	9-10 oz-eq.	10-11 oz-eq.
Meat & Beans	4 oz-eq.	5 oz-eq.	5-5.5 oz-eq.	5.5-6.5 oz-eq.	6.5-7 oz-eq.	7-7.5 oz-eq.	7-7.5 oz-eq.	7.5-8 oz-eq.
Milk	2-3 c.	3 c.	3 c.	3 c.	3 c.	3 c.	3 c.	3 c.
Healthy Oils	4 tsp.	5 tsp.	5 tsp.	6 tsp.	6 tsp.	7 tsp.	8 tsp.	8 tsp.

Day One

FOOD CHOICES
Breakfast: _____   Lunch: _____

Dinner: _____   Snacks: _____

Group	Fruits	Vegetables	Grains	Meat & Beans	Milk	Oils
Goal Amount						
Estimate Your Total						
Increase ⇧ or Decrease ⇩ ?						

PHYSICAL ACTIVITY   SPIRITUAL ACTIVITY

Description: _____   Description: _____

Steps/Miles/Minutes: _____   _____

Day Two

FOOD CHOICES
Breakfast: _____   Lunch: _____

Dinner: _____   Snacks: _____

Group	Fruits	Vegetables	Grains	Meat & Beans	Milk	Oils
Goal Amount						
Estimate Your Total						
Increase ⇧ or Decrease ⇩ ?						

PHYSICAL ACTIVITY   SPIRITUAL ACTIVITY

Description: _____   Description: _____

Steps/Miles/Minutes: _____   _____

Day Three

FOOD CHOICES
Breakfast: _____   Lunch: _____

Dinner: _____   Snacks: _____

Group	Fruits	Vegetables	Grains	Meat & Beans	Milk	Oils
Goal Amount						
Estimate Your Total						
Increase ⇧ or Decrease ⇩ ?						

PHYSICAL ACTIVITY   SPIRITUAL ACTIVITY

Description: _____   Description: _____

Steps/Miles/Minutes: _____

Day Four

FOOD CHOICES

Breakfast: _____ Lunch: _____

Dinner: _____ Snacks: _____

Group	Fruits	Vegetables	Grains	Meat & Beans	Milk	Oils
Goal Amount						
Estimate Your Total						
Increase ⇧ or Decrease ⇩ ?						

PHYSICAL ACTIVITY

Description: _____

Steps/Miles/Minutes: _____

SPIRITUAL ACTIVITY

Description: _____

_____

Day Five

FOOD CHOICES

Breakfast: _____ Lunch: _____

Dinner: _____ Snacks: _____

Group	Fruits	Vegetables	Grains	Meat & Beans	Milk	Oils
Goal Amount						
Estimate Your Total						
Increase ⇧ or Decrease ⇩ ?						

PHYSICAL ACTIVITY

Description: _____

Steps/Miles/Minutes: _____

SPIRITUAL ACTIVITY

Description: _____

_____

Day Six

FOOD CHOICES

Breakfast: _____ Lunch: _____

Dinner: _____ Snacks: _____

Group	Fruits	Vegetables	Grains	Meat & Beans	Milk	Oils
Goal Amount						
Estimate Your Total						
Increase ⇧ or Decrease ⇩ ?						

PHYSICAL ACTIVITY

Description: _____

Steps/Miles/Minutes: _____

SPIRITUAL ACTIVITY

Description: _____

_____

Day Seven

FOOD CHOICES

Breakfast: _____ Lunch: _____

Dinner: _____ Snacks: _____

Group	Fruits	Vegetables	Grains	Meat & Beans	Milk	Oils
Goal Amount						
Estimate Your Total						
Increase ⇧ or Decrease ⇩ ?						

PHYSICAL ACTIVITY

Description: _____

Steps/Miles/Minutes: _____

SPIRITUAL ACTIVITY

Description: _____

_____

Live It Tracker

Name: _____ My week at a glance: ☐ Great ☐ So-so ☐ Not so great

Date: _____ Week #: _____ Calorie Range: _____ My food goal for next week: _____

Activity Level: None, < 30 min/day, 30-60 min/day, 60+ min/day My activity goal for next week: _____

Scripture Memory Verse: _____

RECOMMENDED DAILY AMOUNT OF FOOD FROM EACH GROUP

Group	Daily Calories							
	1300-1400	1500-1600	1700-1800	1900-2000	2100-2200	2300-2400	2500-2600	2700-2800
Fruits	1.5-2 c.	1.5-2 c.	1.5-2 c.	2-2.5 c.	2-2.5 c.	2.5-3.5 c.	3.5-4.5 c.	3.5-4.5 c.
Vegetables	1.5-2 c.	2-2.5 c.	2.5-3 c.	2.5-3 c.	3-3.5 c.	3.5-4.5 c.	4.5-5 c.	4.5-5 c.
Grains	5 oz-eq.	5-6 oz-eq.	6-7 oz-eq.	6-7 oz-eq.	7-8 oz-eq.	8-9 oz-eq.	9-10 oz-eq.	10-11 oz-eq.
Meat & Beans	4 oz-eq.	5 oz-eq.	5-5.5 oz-eq.	5.5-6.5 oz-eq.	6.5-7 oz-eq.	7-7.5 oz-eq.	7-7.5 oz-eq.	7.5-8 oz-eq.
Milk	2-3 c.	3 c.	3 c.	3 c.	3 c.	3 c.	3 c.	3 c.
Healthy Oils	4 tsp.	5 tsp.	5 tsp.	6 tsp.	6 tsp.	7 tsp.	8 tsp.	8 tsp.

Day One

FOOD CHOICES

Breakfast: _____ Lunch: _____

Dinner: _____ Snacks: _____

Group	Fruits	Vegetables	Grains	Meat & Beans	Milk	Oils
Goal Amount						
Estimate Your Total						
Increase ⇧ or Decrease ⇩ ?						

PHYSICAL ACTIVITY **SPIRITUAL ACTIVITY**

Description: _____ Description: _____

Steps/Miles/Minutes: _____

Day Two

FOOD CHOICES

Breakfast: _____ Lunch: _____

Dinner: _____ Snacks: _____

Group	Fruits	Vegetables	Grains	Meat & Beans	Milk	Oils
Goal Amount						
Estimate Your Total						
Increase ⇧ or Decrease ⇩ ?						

PHYSICAL ACTIVITY **SPIRITUAL ACTIVITY**

Description: _____ Description: _____

Steps/Miles/Minutes: _____

Day Three

FOOD CHOICES

Breakfast: _____ Lunch: _____

Dinner: _____ Snacks: _____

Group	Fruits	Vegetables	Grains	Meat & Beans	Milk	Oils
Goal Amount						
Estimate Your Total						
Increase ⇧ or Decrease ⇩ ?						

PHYSICAL ACTIVITY **SPIRITUAL ACTIVITY**

Description: _____ Description: _____

Steps/Miles/Minutes: _____

Day Four

FOOD CHOICES

Breakfast: _____ Lunch: _____

Dinner: _____ Snacks: _____

Group	Fruits	Vegetables	Grains	Meat & Beans	Milk	Oils
Goal Amount						
Estimate Your Total						
Increase ⇧ or Decrease ⇩ ?						

PHYSICAL ACTIVITY

Description: _____

Steps/Miles/Minutes: _____

SPIRITUAL ACTIVITY

Description: _____

_____

Day Five

FOOD CHOICES

Breakfast: _____ Lunch: _____

Dinner: _____ Snacks: _____

Group	Fruits	Vegetables	Grains	Meat & Beans	Milk	Oils
Goal Amount						
Estimate Your Total						
Increase ⇧ or Decrease ⇩ ?						

PHYSICAL ACTIVITY

Description: _____

Steps/Miles/Minutes: _____

SPIRITUAL ACTIVITY

Description: _____

_____

Day Six

FOOD CHOICES

Breakfast: _____ Lunch: _____

Dinner: _____ Snacks: _____

Group	Fruits	Vegetables	Grains	Meat & Beans	Milk	Oils
Goal Amount						
Estimate Your Total						
Increase ⇧ or Decrease ⇩ ?						

PHYSICAL ACTIVITY

Description: _____

Steps/Miles/Minutes: _____

SPIRITUAL ACTIVITY

Description: _____

_____

Day Seven

FOOD CHOICES

Breakfast: _____ Lunch: _____

Dinner: _____ Snacks: _____

Group	Fruits	Vegetables	Grains	Meat & Beans	Milk	Oils
Goal Amount						
Estimate Your Total						
Increase ⇧ or Decrease ⇩ ?						

PHYSICAL ACTIVITY

Description: _____

Steps/Miles/Minutes: _____

SPIRITUAL ACTIVITY

Description: _____

_____

Live It Tracker

Name: _____ My week at a glance: ☐ Great ☐ So-so ☐ Not so great

Date: _____ Week #: _____ Calorie Range: _____ My food goal for next week: _____

Activity Level: None, < 30 min/day, 30-60 min/day, 60+ min/day   My activity goal for next week: _____

Scripture Memory Verse: _____

RECOMMENDED DAILY AMOUNT OF FOOD FROM EACH GROUP

Group	Daily Calories							
	1300-1400	1500-1600	1700-1800	1900-2000	2100-2200	2300-2400	2500-2600	2700-2800
Fruits	1.5-2 c.	1.5-2 c.	1.5-2 c.	2-2.5 c.	2-2.5 c.	2.5-3.5 c.	3.5-4.5 c.	3.5-4.5 c.
Vegetables	1.5-2 c.	2-2.5 c.	2.5-3 c.	2.5-3 c.	3-3.5 c.	3.5-4.5 c.	4.5-5 c.	4.5-5 c.
Grains	5 oz-eq.	5-6 oz-eq.	6-7 oz-eq.	6-7 oz-eq.	7-8 oz-eq.	8-9 oz-eq.	9-10 oz-eq.	10-11 oz-eq.
Meat & Beans	4 oz-eq.	5 oz-eq.	5-5.5 oz-eq.	5.5-6.5 oz-eq.	6.5-7 oz-eq.	7-7.5 oz-eq.	7-7.5 oz-eq.	7.5-8 oz-eq.
Milk	2-3 c.	3 c.	3 c.	3 c.	3 c.	3 c.	3 c.	3 c.
Healthy Oils	4 tsp.	5 tsp.	5 tsp.	6 tsp.	6 tsp.	7 tsp.	8 tsp.	8 tsp.

Day One

FOOD CHOICES

Breakfast: _____ Lunch: _____

Dinner: _____ Snacks: _____

Group	Fruits	Vegetables	Grains	Meat & Beans	Milk	Oils
Goal Amount						
Estimate Your Total						
Increase ⬆ or Decrease ⬇ ?						

PHYSICAL ACTIVITY   **SPIRITUAL ACTIVITY**

Description: _____ Description: _____

Steps/Miles/Minutes: _____ _____

Day Two

FOOD CHOICES

Breakfast: _____ Lunch: _____

Dinner: _____ Snacks: _____

Group	Fruits	Vegetables	Grains	Meat & Beans	Milk	Oils
Goal Amount						
Estimate Your Total						
Increase ⬆ or Decrease ⬇ ?						

PHYSICAL ACTIVITY   **SPIRITUAL ACTIVITY**

Description: _____ Description: _____

Steps/Miles/Minutes: _____ _____

Day Three

FOOD CHOICES

Breakfast: _____ Lunch: _____

Dinner: _____ Snacks: _____

Group	Fruits	Vegetables	Grains	Meat & Beans	Milk	Oils
Goal Amount						
Estimate Your Total						
Increase ⬆ or Decrease ⬇ ?						

PHYSICAL ACTIVITY   **SPIRITUAL ACTIVITY**

Description: _____ Description: _____

Steps/Miles/Minutes: _____ _____

Day Four

FOOD CHOICES

Breakfast: _____ Lunch: _____

Dinner: _____ Snacks: _____

Group	Fruits	Vegetables	Grains	Meat & Beans	Milk	Oils
Goal Amount						
Estimate Your Total						
Increase ⬆ or Decrease ⬇ ?						

PHYSICAL ACTIVITY

Description: _____

Steps/Miles/Minutes: _____

SPIRITUAL ACTIVITY

Description: _____

_____

Day Five

FOOD CHOICES

Breakfast: _____ Lunch: _____

Dinner: _____ Snacks: _____

Group	Fruits	Vegetables	Grains	Meat & Beans	Milk	Oils
Goal Amount						
Estimate Your Total						
Increase ⬆ or Decrease ⬇ ?						

PHYSICAL ACTIVITY

Description: _____

Steps/Miles/Minutes: _____

SPIRITUAL ACTIVITY

Description: _____

_____

Day Six

FOOD CHOICES

Breakfast: _____ Lunch: _____

Dinner: _____ Snacks: _____

Group	Fruits	Vegetables	Grains	Meat & Beans	Milk	Oils
Goal Amount						
Estimate Your Total						
Increase ⬆ or Decrease ⬇ ?						

PHYSICAL ACTIVITY

Description: _____

Steps/Miles/Minutes: _____

SPIRITUAL ACTIVITY

Description: _____

_____

Day Seven

FOOD CHOICES

Breakfast: _____ Lunch: _____

Dinner: _____ Snacks: _____

Group	Fruits	Vegetables	Grains	Meat & Beans	Milk	Oils
Goal Amount						
Estimate Your Total						
Increase ⬆ or Decrease ⬇ ?						

PHYSICAL ACTIVITY

Description: _____

Steps/Miles/Minutes: _____

SPIRITUAL ACTIVITY

Description: _____

_____

contributors

Diane Bagby
Houston, Texas

June Chapko
San Antonio, Texas

Jim Clayton
Lenoir City, Tennessee

Elizabeth Crews
Chula Vista, California

Betha Jean Cunningham
San Angelo, Texas

Erin DuBroc
Houston, Texas

Vicki Heath
North Charleston,
South Carolina

Claudia Korff
Houston, Texas

Barb Lee
Normal, Illinois

Carole Lewis
Houston, Texas

Barbara Lukies
Farmborough Heights,
NSW, Australia

Marca MacGregor
Summerville, South Carolina

Judy Marshall
Gilmer, Texas

Dee Matthews
Sugar Land, Texas

Martha Rogers
Houston, Texas

Bev Schwind
Fairfield Glade, Tennessee

David Self
Houston, Texas

Becky Sims
Hilliars, Ohio

Karrie Smyth
Brandon, Manitoba, Canada

Carol Van Atta
Troutdale, Oregon

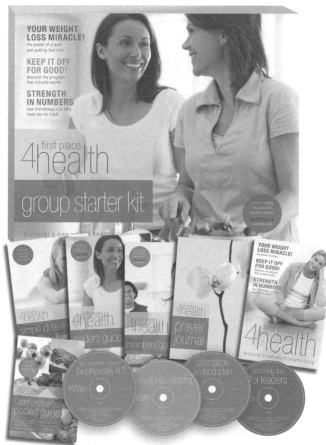
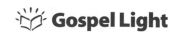

first place 4health
discover a new way to healthy living

Change Your Life Forever by Putting Christ First!

Start Today with These First Place 4 Health Bible Studies

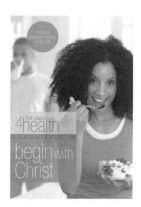

Begin with Christ
The first in a new series of Bible studies for the First Place 4 Health program, *Begin with Christ* will help members focus on surrendering to God.

ISBN 10-digit: 08307.45181
ISBN 13-digit: 978.08307.45180

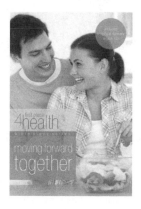

Moving Forward Together
Give participants new inspiration to focus on the journey of following Christ and living according to His guidelines.

ISBN 10-digit: 08307.45203
ISBN 13-digit: 978.08307.45203

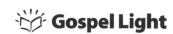 **Gospel Light**